MEET
YOURSELF

MEET
YOURSELF

De-addict yourself from
gadgets today using YOGA.

Yog will change your life

Palak Garg

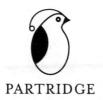

PARTRIDGE

To order additional copies of this book, contact
Partridge India
000 800 10062 62
orders.india@partridgepublishing.com

www.partridgepublishing.com/india

Contents

Acknowledgements

I owe a debt of gratitude to my mom; thank you for believing in me, encouraging me in all of my pursuits, and inspiring me to follow my thoughts.

To my adorable father, a great self-made entrepreneur, for unflinching financial support.

To Dr Sumer Singh, my principal, who has succeeded in getting our institution, The Daly College, recognized globally and getting us fair opportunities.

To Mrs Asma Ansari, Dean CIE, for her very constructive criticism and careful attention paid at my performances.

To Mr Khalid Syyed, HOD, business studies, for modeling great teaching and for furthering my thinking about studying business.

My yoga guru, Pundit Radheshyam Mishra, who is fiercely committed in spreading yoga, for being my data bank.

To my yoga guru, Mrs Dipti Gami, for introducing me to myself, and always being there as a mentor for me.

To my Yoga guru, Veda Chaitanya (Ajay Sir), for introducing me to wider and international aspects of yoga, and for offering his professional guidance whenever I require him.

To Mrs Anju Bindal, who has been the backbone of my language and who has offered her incredible editing expertise every time.

To Mrs Anita Motwani, my math teacher, who has always boosted my confidence.

To my yoga friends, Dr Karthik Kasyap, Ms Neha Khanuja, and Mr Vijay Soni for supporting me at all times, at times of storms too, and lighting the flame of yogic way of living and thinking within me.

To my PR and branding manager, Mrs Vatsala Garg, whose contributions cannot be ignored.

To my yoga photographer, great artist, Mr Vivek Samaiya, for capturing the real essence.

My family members, Maa, Dada, Nana, Gudia Maasi, Abhishek Uncle, Khushboo Mami, Meenakshi Aunty for tolerating stubborn me as I am.

Minakshi Mangal, my best friend, needs a special mention in this for always keeping her arms open for me and being my corner of support and understanding.

My bestest buddies Divija, Sanaya, Dia, Palash, Anisha, Keshav, Tejasvee, Ishita, and Nehal, I can't imagine days without you guys.

To my nanny, Sunita Aunty, for raising me like her own daughter.

My cute young family, my life, Aaryan, Khwaish, Ayaan, Aanya, Ansh, Riaan, Vipul, Anish, Kanishk, Pranav, Aarav, and Vinnie, love you all to the moon and back. This research I dedicate to you all.

To the Publishing, Technical and Editorial team of Patridge Publishing, without your patience and cooperation, this compiling of my research would not have been possible.

Disclaimer

Some names and identifying details have been changed to protect the privacy of many individuals. I advise readers to take full responsibility for their safety and know their limits. Before practicing the skills described in this book, be sure you do not take risks beyond your level of experience, aptitude, training, and comfort level.

The content of this book is solely my opinion based on my research, and does not in any way intend to contradict or deny other's opinions or thinking.

About the Author

Born in the year 1999, Palak was the first child to her industrialist parents. Born and brought up in Central India, she has an extraordinary memory and logical reasoning according to her mother.

Currently finishing off her high school in grade twelve, she is an incredible athlete and has been winning various accolades for the same for the last eight years now. She is a strongly academically inclined girl and has been winning awards for her credentials. Serving in the prefectorial board of her school, she has been representing her school in on-screen quiz contests, round square conferences, and various model United Nations in renowned institutions throughout the globe.

She is a very ambitious girl who wants to graduate from her ideal college in business management, and aspires to become an entrepreneur in the future. At such a young age, she is a certified international yoga instructor, and wishes to spread it's aspects in modern lives globally. She's been researching on the topic 'causes of gadget addiction' deeply and has been trying to eradicate this evil phenomenon through the calming practise of yoga. After an in depth analysis of various methods and relating yoga to every aspect of gadgets, she finally came up and shared her views with such a large audience through writing.

Writing a book on de-addiction would have been impossible without thinking like an addict. Thankfully, this girl had the potential to think from that perspective and produce such a justified piece.

Preface

My mother always cautioned me about this dangerous disorder of gadget addiction. She cribbed me constantly for giving up my phone and limited my hours online. I have always grown up wondering as a child what exactly gadget addiction is, and why is it such a detrimental phenomenon for me or for any individual for that matter.

This topic has long been my research topic, and I have tried to link it with every aspect of my life in order to compare its causes, effects, and significance in my life. Whilst noticing my own technological usage, I realised the influence of my practise of yoga on my online behavioral issues. Yoga has always been a significant part of my life and has helped me to almost totally eradicate the consumption of electronic devices. Not only this, it has played a major role in minimizing the effects of daily usage of some technical gadgets. Through this calming practise, de-addiction can be extremely easy and very helpful in the long run. Yoga is one of the most relaxing and stress-relieving practises, which has no possible drawbacks, and can help any human being to improve both mind and body.

In this generation, I strongly feel that it is an utmost necessity for each of us to lessen our dependence on these technological gadgets in order to avoid getting overly addicted and then facing numerous deleterious effects. Everyone must understand that a few minutes spent on improving your mind and body is much more beneficial than wasting hours and hours on destructive tools. Personally, even I never understood how negatively my laptop or my mobile was influencing me, but once my practise of constantly checking updates decreased, I realised how I was improving my life and focusing on things that actually matter. So one never admits about the problem, but it's there, and it is better to avoid it.

Chapter 1

YOU NEED HELP

Mom was giving me the usual everyday lecture cautioning me about the dangerous disorder of gadget addiction and cribbing constantly for giving up my phone and limit my hours online, as she felt gadgets were causing too many harms to my performance and my behaviour. But as usual, her impactless lectures went in one ear and came straight out of the other. All this crying and nagging of hers made me feel stupid about her, and rather increased my dependency on gadgets.

One day, my mom entered my room in morning to wake me up, but I was already awake as my social media updates provided me a reason to get out of bed every day. I waited for the usual lecture, but to my relief, it never came. I believe my insincerity toward her attitude had finally made her realise that talking about cons and pros of gadget was a sheer waste of time to a gadget freak like me. She slammed the door close and went, but that began to open the doors in my brain. That made me realise that maybe she is sick of my neglection, and maybe she had accepted she has failed to change me.

I started to imagine that Mom was a gadget lover, and spent all her time on social media without paying attention to her daily chores, our meals, our laundry, groceries, etc. One day, during my vacations, Mom kept chatting with friends and family members all the time and didn't even care to pay attention that I had just entered home. I noticed that her indulgence into gadgets led to the breads burning in kitchen, the milk boiling out of the saucepan, my younger brother shouting on top if his voice when he couldn't find his school uniform, my father screaming from toilet to switch on the water motor, but she did not seem to care a bit and left it all unattended. Then suddenly, my thoughts wandered to my father, and I started thinking about his lifestyle.

I started portraying him with his laptop on his lap, lying in bed without going to office, and office staff is calling him several times, but he is not attending any calls. And when my mother asks him for her usual monthly household expenditure money, he says, 'I have none.'

That very thought shivered me. Those very words 'no money' made me sink with the belief I always carried that gadgets were useful every time. I started thinking how can one earn money when one is only confined to gadgets all the time? How would my mother have raised me with gadgets in her hand? These questions puzzled me to bits. However, after reading this example, every gadget freak will try to console himself that he will never let his gadget usage reach up that stage, but in reality, neither of us can stop ourselves.

Seeing my parents fulfill their responsibilities without any excuses, and being so tolerant toward us, suddenly hit me with the guilt of what I had been doing for all those years. With those ingenious excuses for my obsession for smart devices, how painful it would have been for my parents to see a happy, intelligent, gentle, and considerate child to change into an aggressive violent short-tempered devil.

'I will stay away' were the exact words pondering in my mind when I accepted the fact and regretted in front of my mother. However, her expression was more disappointing than the usual daily lectures. The look clearly stated that she believed I am trying to convince her for an outing with my friends, or demanding a signature on a worksheet in which I have scored a grade *C*. Her look and expression were totally justified because she had seen me delivering thousands of failed promises of fixing on-screen time with gadgets earlier too. I could sense her feeling—how helpless she found herself to be in making me realise that my gadget addiction is the cause of all the problems.

Till now, I had been disowning all her attempts to cope up with me. But now, it had started a reaction inside me that I hoped to tell my mom, 'Mom, you will see this happen.' I was sensing a feeling of independence. Independence from the evil trap of smart devices! Now I needed help.

Now, I no longer feel ashamed of my mother's reliance on me or my younger brother for any technical help with gadgets, and now I understand my grandfather telling me stories of how Doordarshan (Indian television channel), radio, and trunk call booking (phone call booking made to speak to a distant person) were the only resorts for his generation with just one or two buttons to operate those mechanisms. My grandparents call those days with sheer joy 'those good old days.'

Chapter 2

WHAT IS GADGET ADDICTION?

The first inventors of electronics were considered the 'Gods' for the convenience and time-saving they brought for mankind. But irony of the fact is that now, I have to come forward and explain my friends how electronics have nothing but an inconvenience and have taken away a lot of precious time away from mankind.

Technology has been extremely beneficial in one way and so incredibly harmful in another. To spread my word and harms of gadgets with the help of gadgets only is again bone crushing. It takes every piece of energy to make an addict realise that he has fallen in a trap that he cannot very easily escape till the time he keeps convincing himself that he is in control of himself. In fact, even if the addict realises, to some extent, he will keep saying 'Okay! I agree that I need to stop using too many devices for my own sake, but not today, or let me play for one last time.'

Believe me, there will be no last time! In some cases, even if he realises he is an addict, he will buy a book on de-addiction or read an article like this to keep in his mind that there were some remedy when he needed it. Maybe not now.

Don't our adrenaline levels go up after we get to know that someone liked our profile picture on Facebook or followed us on Instagram? Don't we regain our good cheer when we spot our iPhones or iPads fully charged? Don't we find our concentration suffering and our grades falling consistently from straight *A*'s because of constantly gawking at the screens? If your answer to any one of these questions is a 'Yes,' the chances are that we teenagers have become yet another victim of gadget addiction.

Gadget addiction is one of the most common kinds of addictions found in today's youth, in which it becomes impossible for an individual to free himself or herself from the shackles of any particular product; and in this scenario, the ever-growing technology, or the most fascinating source for some of us, the Internet.

Gadget addiction is considered a real mental disorder in many different countries. Any of us who was born after 1990 has never known life without the Internet and mobile communication. Those of us who are presently growing up with cell phones and interactive video games can't imagine living without them.

A babysitter needs a television to make the child have food, a teenager in today's era needs applications like Facebook and Whatsapp to be updated with the world and for social status, a housewife needs online shopping websites for ordering different things. The reasons we use technology and electronic gadgets for are not that significant in proportion to the role of gadgets in our lives. The teenagers are especially becoming slaves to these gadgets, and crave for recharging their dying batteries more than for food after skipping a meal.

We use gadgets for things which could easily be done without our overdependence on these addictive devices.

Once we start to consume these tools, we are always urge driven and want more of them. This cycle continues, and we are attracted to utilise more of these gadgets. Once we start using these devices so frequently that we actually lose count of our actions, it becomes very difficult for us to let go of our habit of using tech-gadgets for everything we do; we never realise that our desire of using electronic devices has gradually been converted into gadget addiction. In fact, these technologies can become so all-consuming that susceptible individuals showcase very complex addictive properties. When we are not online, we are thinking about being online. We stay up all night, leading to different mental and health-related issues. Certain kinds of video games have proven to trigger a neurological response in all age groups of children.

Those of us who are highly addicted to our mobile phones, and need it to carry every petty activity of our lives, develop a kind of phobia, which is well known as nomophobia. In nomophobia, a person is afraid of leaving his or her phone unattended.

Gadget addiction, like any other addiction, severely debilitates our capacities for achieving our dreams, and in the whole process, transforms us into lazy, uninterested individuals.

All individuals do exhibit certain characteristics, which can be understood as developing addiction. Those certain characteristics are:

> If we exhibit complete lack of interest in other activities—even our favorite ones like going for a movie or a game of football

▌ If we become argumentative whenever the topic of excess gadget time is brought up. We might also become exceedingly offensive or defensive in our arguments and fail to view the whole issue.

▌ If we becomes excessively despondent when we are unable to access our online accounts and gain good cheer once we are able to

▌ If we start lying to our parents about our gadget utilization timings in an attempt to delude them from reality

▌ If we get anxious and irritable if we don't have our favourite electronic gadgets with us

The technology continues to connect countries and communities, but chooses to neglect how it is also responsible for disturbing our planet.

It is merely isolating us and pushing each one of us into lonely, colorless lives.

Chapter 3

THOSE WHO DON'T OVERCOME THEIR FEARS

We need it right now, but the fear instilled in us of not having enough willpower and desire to de-addict does not allow us to accept that we need to de-addict now. It is an utmost necessity to de-addict now, not tomorrow or day after. Even if we, as individuals, overcome our fears, we ponder about why is there a need to de-addict today. There's a life ahead! Let me prove my presence to my peers on social media today for the last time.

We keep postponing for umpteen number of times as possible. The addiction makes us feel what will we do without these devices? How will we stay in touch? How will our peers connect to us? But in reality, contrary to our beliefs, the social media is actually making us anti-social. We are in a fake connection with world with no actual connect with even our close family members.

Let's see the number of deaths due to any kind of addiction on the globe in a day.

Alcohol xxx
Drugs xx

Tobacco xxxx
Technology????
(by 2025)

How can technology cause deaths? It's not regarded as a disease in itself! This is due to the technology not having any obvious effects on our health. But what is accountable for maximum number of suicides? Suicides due to depression, emptiness, stress of not performing well, regression, betrayal, jealousy, competition, relationship, and the list of psychological hurts is endless. Where do all these feelings generate from? Each one reading this will have a true answer to this in his/her heart somewhere. Maybe we can't put up in words or accept the crux of the problem.

1. A young boy of seven years tried to win the second level of certain game, but despite his several hours and days of attempts, he could not succeed. He ended his life miserably. Was it even worth it?

2. Two friends of age fourteen attended a theme party. One posted few pictures tagging her friend. Unfortunately, pictures of the tagged friend got thirty-eight more likes than hers. She felt she had lost a battle. Did she really?

3. A 19-year-old boy posted the pictures of his graduation ceremony. He mentioned one of his girl classmate as his mentor and greatest support in class twelfth. His girlfriend saw and started abusing him on the same media. She felt betrayed! Was it actually betrayal? Have relationships become so fragile due to so many things happening around?

4. A 17-year-old girl had four other girls in her group. Other four girls had crush at some point. This girl started feeling like she was left behind in the race. She made friends on most active media to win. She started sharing all her details, her travelling plans, her status, etc., not knowing who is she sharing the details with actually. And she was raped by this same guy at her own residence! Was she actually looking for this kind of relationship?

5. To my shock, a divorcee of forty-four years was trying to look for her soulmate on online matrimonial portals. She accepted a request of a profile telling about himself as a doctor in the US. The woman was overwhelmed with a great match. They both started having conversations. After two and half months, man announced, 'Hurray! Got the visa sanctioned. I am coming to India, we will marry after twenty days.' In these twenty days, he kept posting the pictures of things he said he is shopping for his would-be wife. Almost one hundred things were claimed to be bought for his lady. Then came the day of his coming to India. The lady got a call, there was a lady on other end declaring that Mr X is stopped by the customs in Delhi for carrying the stuff worth millions. And the would-be bride will have to pay two lacks to take him out from here. Though in dilemma, but the female of forty-four thought of helping her love and deposited two lacks in the account no stated by the phone call and kept trying the nan's phone number. To her surprise, the phone was switched off and matrimonial profile no

more existed! A one-time divorcee was filled with emptiness and thoughts of ending her life.

6. A 20-year-old boy sensed an attraction between a boy and a girl of his own batch, and registered a fake profile by the boy's name and started approaching the girl, proposed to her, and exchanged some intimate conversation asking the girl to post her pictures. The girl also, without thinking, did so as she was committed to the relationship. Then after a flash trade of four months, she ended up committing suicide because the boy was blackmailing her with the screenshots of previous conversations they had exchanged.

7. A 13-year-old boy was caught watching porn sites by his 18-year-old brother. The young boy jumped down immediately from his balcony! Was this the only embarrassment caused?

8. An 8-year-old boy, while returning from school with his chauffer, demanded to stop at a store. When he returned, he was holding a cigarette with great style. This was later brought into the notice of his father by the chauffer. On asking the boy that what was he trying to do, he answered he had seen his favorite cartoon character Popeye carrying a pipe in his mouth permanently, though there are warnings written at those scenes that smoking is injurious to health. But are all these cautionary communications effective? Even the seat belts are made compulsory, but we are aware of the facts that how many lives are being saved by introduction of the precaution.

They are merely not examples, but evidences of how over usage, over reliability, and total dependency on technology have paralysed our senses and have started making us believe that fake is real. Not only this, the biggest disaster is that 8 per cent of the world's population is suffering from gadget addiction, and all intelligent addicts all over the world are aware of the facts. The violence, drugs, and sex available on social media are affecting the behaviour of the youth.

Chapter 4

PARENTS BRIBE

A 3-year-old boy named Ansh was running away from his mother, as she was trying to feed him. Both of them were running around the house. When the mother, who was trying to chase Ansh, had to stop him, she gave him her iPad to play X game; and to her satisfaction, he sat down and finally started having food.

But did the mother realise that she had introduced the thought of getting iPad as a reward in the boy's mind for finishing his food? She started programming the little child's mind by making him believe that he must expect a little reward if he completes his meal without running around. Because of her, didn't Ansh started finding pleasure in materialistic objects/flashy coloured screens, or fast moving cars and bikes seen in virtual games? Didn't he resort to the other evil-violence?

The fact is that parents try to reward or bribe children with technology themselves, then put in all their energy to unhook them! In order to fill the emptiness created by their own absence due to the modern society pressures, parents tend to fill it with more screen hours. But in contrast to their thinking, they are actually making children irritable and insecure. They worsen the situation by being overly protective about their children, and introducing them to automation or labour-saving devices. They, in turn, eliminate the habit of thinking and solving using their respective brains. A parent's education is also required to solve the problem unless who cannot afford these dubious pleasures.

Sarah, of twelve years, returned from school and immediately opened her elder sister's laptop. Her sister questioned her need to use her laptop. Sarah replied that she had to finish a project in social studies to write and draw on traffic rules. This kind of unawareness rings a bell in us that children who travel for long kilometres to their schools and classes don't know basic traffic rules, and can't visualize a project or a drawing or an essay without the Internet. They find it difficult to think about basic subjects. They have lost interest in creating, finding out, or talking about various subjects.

As they've discovered exciting new area of finding out things in seconds on the Internet, their lack of interest has become very acute. They just want to finish up the project or assignment with the help of Internet. They don't enjoy their work, and instead, find their school assignment distressing.

The truth is no parents encourage their children to revert to gadgets, but they do not educate them either. It is not only a parent's desire, but also the duty of every parent to educate their children with the dangers of life, not merely make them aware of dangers of Internet and leave them to choose.

If suppose your son decided to bang his thumb with a hammer or jump off the roof or immerse his hand in boiling water, would you just point out that action's pros and cons, or would you actually make sure that he doesn't do so?

Yagya, of age seventeen, had a habit of biting nails since she was two, and despite her strong desire to give up the habit, she failed! That was merely a habit as it was physical, but bonding with gadgets is addiction as it exists simply in mind. Parents should teach the true implication of the difference between habit and addiction before arises a day, and children become old enough to look straight into your eyes and deny your opinion point-blank.

I recollect an incident of Naina, a girl of sixteen years, who was seen spending all her time on Snapchat, which is a live photo-sharing portal. Despite all futile attempts of understanding how risky it can be at times for a teenager like her, she believed, 'My parents keep lecturing me all the time, so I use Snapchat to rebel against them.' She became rebel against the people who loved her the most!

Naina, in just few days, got restrigated from school, as she was found carrying mobile secretly in her school bag. Everyone thought that she will definitely feel ashamed by this incident and change. But she said, 'Either way, my problems in this school are finally over.' Her response is of course astonishing! Is today's youth aware where this attitude of ours will take us?

Chapter 5

WEIGHT GAIN IS SURE

The first and the foremost consequence of over utilisation of gadgets is that electronic devices turn us into couch potatoes, thereby making us extremely lazy and resulting in obesity. Obesity is on the rise because of gadget addiction, and industry experts warn us of an unhealthy future citing lack of activity. Both adults and children cannot do without gadgets. Physical activity has reduced significantly since Internet came into being. We are spending more time indoors than outdoors. Yes! Its games and different engaging applications have become quite popular amongst us, and hence, they are turning us into obese human beings.

A large number of us are also becoming obese due to constantly snacking on junk food, while being totally engaged with different gadgets. We never realise, but we tend to overeat when we are engaged with an engrossing gadget. Intake of carbonated drinks is highest when we tend to spend our times online either chatting or watching movies.

Sujoy, was a 12-year-old boy, but was pot bellied as much a man of 60 years old. Neither was he born overweight nor was he like this two years before. The belly of this size was just a gain of two years from the time he had stopped playing tennis and swimming.

Gadgets, or any electronic devices, are the prime causes of obesity, laziness, dullness, inactiveness, etc. A gadget lover avoids all activities when he is with a device, especially sports and school lessons. The energy stored and zest for device makes food more interesting, and you fall in the tendency to eat larger meals and also start picking up and eating junk between main meals, while watching or playing with a device. The little monster inside keeps saying eat, eat, and eat! We believe food is more enjoyable with a device. Obviously, this hunger is not physical, but only mental. Body is incapable of craving for food. The cravings can only be experienced through brain.

Perhaps those young addicts who are thin and lean tend to take it for granted. They believe any amount of eating will however cast no effect on them. The energy generated due to this overeating remains unexhausted by the body. That energy then demands further eating, which makes you feel physically worse and results into short temper, mood swings, frustration, and eventually, that becomes your permanent nature.

Smartphone revolution has taken gadget addiction to the next level. When we have everything we require one click away, we are bound to becoming inactive and lead extremely sedentary lifestyles. This results in us becoming lazy and obese. Many psychologists and psychiatrists have voiced their opinions regarding this issue, and have claimed 'smartphones addiction is not going to be an easy tackle in the future.'

Blues of electronic devices before bedtime could mess up our sleep patterns more profoundly than we ever realise. We take longer time to fall asleep and spend less time relaxing. This irregularity in our sleeping timings can also result in circadian rhythm sleeping disorder. In this, we have problems in the timings of when we sleep and when we are awake. Excessive use of electronics can disrupt our sleeping patterns and hinder our sleeping cycles. This persistent lack of sleep could be associated with dangerous health related issues such as diabetes.

Chapter 6

SOCIAL ISOLATION

Technological gadgets have posed a deleterious impact on social relationships. Every one of us is so indulged in their gadgets that we have no time to sit with our friends and families and spend some quality time with them. We all prefer to connect with our friends and relatives virtually through text messaging, chatting, etc. rather than meeting them in reality. We may enjoy online relationships using social media sites like Facebook or Twitter, for example, but the difference between these kinds of interactions and interactions with people in the physical world is clearly vast.

The problem, which we've come to face, is that we subtly substitute electronic relationships for physical ones or mistake our electronic relationships for physical ones. We may feel we're connecting effectively with others via the Internet, but too much electronic-relating paradoxically engenders a sense of social isolation.

Every time Jai's (a 17-year-old boy) parents asked for an outing or a family dinner, he denied and said he'll relax at home watching television. Later, when he was going out for his further studies, he himself asked his parents, 'I want to enjoy last evening out for family dinner at my favourite restaurant.' Parents were highly eager and happy to hear this. Unfortunately, what should have been the evening to remember turned into a complete disaster for parents, as Jai was on his cell phone for the entire evening. This ruined attempt of parents made them ponder that he was better at home watching television alone. This addiction had made a youngster like Jai forget to even apologise for ruining his parent's emotions.

You will definitely notice this great disorder while flying too. Once, while I was travelling, beside my seat on right hand corner was sitting a young gadget junkie (maybe of fifteen years). He settled on his seat immediately with his laptop fixed on his tray table and started the loud violent movie, which maybe he had saved thinking he will obtain some genuine pleasure, while watching it only during flight and eating. Without even noticing how other co-passengers were staring, the boy's eyes were fixed at screen while he kept eating constantly and stubbornly fiddling with the wrappers, creating yet another irritating sound. The fellow old aged passenger was trying to close his ears with his hand, but did not complain, thinking the boy will have all the arguments ready like he is within his rights and so on and reflect all his frustration at the helpless old man. Politeness and gratitude were no more basic courteous manners of the young gadget freak.

Not only this, there is also an observation of people using electronic media to make confrontation easier, and have seen more than one relationship falter as a result. People are often uncomfortable with face-to-face confrontation, so it's easy to understand why they'd choose to use the Internet. Precisely because electronic media transmits emotion so poorly compared to in-person interaction, many view it as the perfect way to send difficult messages. It blocks us from registering the negative emotional responses such messages engender, which provides us the illusion we're not really doing any sort of great harm.

Unfortunately, this also usually means that we don't transmit these messages with as much empathy, and often find ourselves sending a different message than we intended, and breeding more confusion than we realise.

Chapter 7

HOW IS MEMORY AFFECTED?

A study from the Kaspersky lab, a cybersecurity firm, says, 'People have become accustomed to using computer devices as an extension of their own brain.' It also describes the rise of what it calls 'digital amnesia' in which people are ready to forget important information in the belief that it can be immediately retrieved from a digital device. There was also a growing trend of keeping personal memories in digital form.

Nowadays, the entire world is so dependent on mobile phones or laptops that this overdependence is affecting their mental health gravely. For petty things, people need their phones and the Internet. Due to this, digital amnesia takes place and negatively impacts the human memory and brain. Psychologists say that reliance on mobile or Internet for every detail is not at all beneficial for us. Pressing buttons continuously hinders our progress, as this way, we never feel like learning anything new. In fact, even if we try to learn or memorize something, it becomes impossible for the brain to store everything as the brain's capacity reduces, as we are too used to finding out everything just a click away.

Because of storing everything on gadgets, it becomes routine for us to neglect every chunk of information and only read it when required. This also weakens our memory, as we are not in the habit of recalling information, which is an efficient way of restoring information permanently in our brains. Passive reading on electronic devices does not create a solid, lasting memory trace in our minds.

Due to overdependence in technology, not only do our minds stop working but also the information that we do have becomes worthless. When we can't learn and store anything in our minds, we don't have anything to contemplate about. Our mind becomes like a vegetable—an object which does not have it's own thinking power. All our functions slow down, and we become very dull and mentally inactive in life. Now, the very little information, which we do have stored in the back of our minds, also becomes useless. This is so because we don't use that knowledge and information anywhere. More than using, we don't apply that particular knowledge in its practical form. We are so engulfed in the electronic world that we don't make optimum use of the little memory left with us. Our minds are always filled about the latest versions of iPhones and Macbooks to ever think about or concentrate on anything else.

A 12-year-old boy, Rahul, was given an assignment in biology to write an essay on how does stress relate to a student's performance. He was supposed to think for himself and wasn't supposed to use any external help to finish this work. However, Rahul went on to search for articles relating to this topic just so that he could run away from the work and receive high praises from his teacher. He copied and pasted the entire article from web. In school, everyone thought that his work was genuine, and he had thorough knowledge about the chapter. His so-called efforts were appreciated by everyone. Till now, nobody knew the actual truth behind his work. During final exams, Rahul suffered tremendously. He didn't remember anything relating to the topic. He was blank during the exam. His brain couldn't recall anything and stopped working completely. After the results were out, he didn't only get bad grades in biology, but he also felt insulted in front of all his classmates and his teacher. Overusage of technology backfired on Rahul's memory really badly, and led him to a hell lot of embarrassment.

Not only is the memory of the brain affected, but also the memories we make can be affected. In today's generation, whenever we travel, we are so engrossed in clicking pictures with our phones and being updated with social media sites that we completely forget about the place and our memories attached to it. We do not seem to care about the happiness the places give up and what they offer, but about how good the pictures come of the places we go to. Only pictures are captured in our minds and not the memories of the places. We never remember the places where we resided or ate or shopped in a particular city. So with dependence on technology, we tend to forget all the memories.

Chapter 8

IT'S ALL IN THE MIND

I remember I kept advising a young addict of twelve years who is also supposedly my junior in my high school, but all my powerful reasons to de-addict proved futile on her, and I started thinking that she is not ready for it, and I'll have to give her some time. One evening, she called me up narrating how she completely got away from the evil trap of technology just in thirty seconds. At 12.30 in midnight, she was surfing through net and casually liked a picture that her favourite English teacher (our headmistress back then) had recently posted. Instantly, there was a message on her mobile, 'You are online so late! No school tomorrow?' That moment, she said, 'I felt so embarrassed that I instantly deleted my profile.'

So this shows that there's no proper time to de-addict, or no threshold to the addiction you are suffering. Everything is in your mind! The problem is mental. When you feel extremely lethargic or suffer from a lack of concentration or confidence, you try to freshen up with your favourite device. You don't understand that the craving itself makes you feel lethargic. The beauty of this addiction is such; the more you are involved with gadgets, the more you are fooled to believe that they are helping you. Your mind is searching for illusory solutions in the service, but this illusion doesn't alter the fact 'fear.' It's like a chicken and an egg coincidence! Did you become lethargic because of gadget, or did gadget took you out of lethargy?

Lily was the highest paid employee of a Robust Company. No one could challenge the presentations she made for defining her marketing strategy, but the irony was that she was unable to do a single word without the help of a device even though she possessed high intelligence, had marketing as her favourite subject, and presentations was not a complication, but a routine for her. This was because making a write up/plan/graph without a device made chills run through her veins. The case became even worse when she refused to her boss to delegate her for any work when WiFi was down.

The real problem like this arises because the device user's brain has been programmed to doubt at user's capability that he/she can't do anything without a device. It all is a mental block, not a reality. We believe that devices are our greatest companions, but irony is that the best friend you trust the most is your enemy, and controls every activity of yours even your hunger.

Anish, a 17-year-old boy was very proud and happy that after waiting for almost a year, his application for 'College Counseling and Application Assisting' for further studies was accepted by the country's most renowned counselor. And after waiting for weeks, then came the day when he was sitting in front of Mr Viral Doshi, the counselor, for a one-to-one counseling session along with his parents. The session went long, and Anish could not control his urge to check the update on his cell phone. Soon, as the session got over and they came outside, his mother asked Anish as to what he thought of the precious advice and suggestion given by Mr Doshi? To her disappointment, she learnt that Anish was so obsessed with not being able to use his smartphone that he had hardly concentrated on any word being said. The mental block, the urge is so strong that an appointment after a wait of almost one year couldn't stop Anish!

Every gadget lover believes that he is different from others, and he uses only for a limited period of time. If any gadget addict does say that, then believe me, he is being incredibly stupid to himself. Perhaps, the gadget addict is preparing himself to accept that he is a coward.

One young teenager of eleven years, after discussing with me casually upon this topic, admitted that he might be nearly an addict, and he took a new year resolution that he will no more be on gadget for games and chats in the commencing year. I can very well recall that this statement was uttered by him in month of September! Irony is that New Year's eve is the most popular time to make productive resolutions, but why postpone it for four more months? Shouldn't it be attempted right now? If you feel an urge to pee, will you postpone it for even four minutes? No.

This fear of staying away from gadgets makes you keep postponing the quit process. This fondness will worsen and worsen and worsen with time! Think of the reason you decide to delay, talk to a friend, write to me. You are definitely not giving up something good. In fact, on the other hand, you are gaining time, confidence, concentration, health, a better vision, and many more marvelous goals. Above all, you gain a self-respect and self-esteem. Open the door and enjoy the bright light.

Chapter 9

ADDICTION? AGE IS NO BAR

Jenny, a 38-year-old lady, was so miserable as if she was suffering from a traumatic situation, or she had lost the most important asset of her life. But to your disguise, she had just cracked her smartphone's screen and was demanding a new device right away. Her husband constantly kept asking her to be reasonable and understand the price paid for owning a smartphone is to accept that the screen can break. However, her impatience was a clear evidence that she was a regular socialite, and all her updates notified her on Whatsapp. Device addiction is not just limited to an age or a gender or a social class.

Uma, a 30-year-old lady, was on a long awaited holiday period on an exotic beach destination with her family after the birth of a younger child. Before leaving from hotel for beach, the family was very, very excited, and kept rushing her and there in order to ensure that they don't miss on anything and do not forget doing any kinds of water sports. When they were finally on the beach, instead of cherishing those moments with family, Uma kept posing for herself and kept posting those selfies immediately on her various social media applications' accounts. This process went on for an hour. At last, she got so tired, frustrated, and bored that she did not even want to talk or play with any of the family members.

Holidays are supposed to be something in which one can relax and not feel any pressure, but Uma was a victim of the social media pressure. Are these the real holidays? Major adults too are irrationally spending 3/4 of their family time with gadgets, and unknowingly and dangerously, they've become dependent on modern devices and cannot survive without them.

Mr. Sujoy, aged 41 years old, was sitting with his 15-months-old daughter on the rear seat of his Car. He was so engrossed in playing a game of cards on his laptop that he did not notice his daughter, who had recently learned how to stand, stood on the seat; and unfortunately, that very moment, the driver pushed the break, and the daughter lost her balance and banged her forehead against the screen fixed at the back of front seat. She started bleeding and was immediately rushed to a hospital where several stiches were put by the doctor to sew the long cut. The young parents have a considerable part to play in getting caught in the trap of gadget addiction, and this evil trap sometimes leads them to even failing to fulfill their basic responsibilities.

The story doesn't end here. Any rational mind will bet that this severe accident would have been enough for Mr Sujoy to delete the game of cards from his laptop, but the unusual thing was that when this whole chaos was over, the first thing Mr Sujoy did was hitting again on that game of cards.

I struck up a conversation with a middle-aged man of around forty-five years who looked like a posh, modern man. To my surprise, he asked a salesman for the cheapest cell phone in the shop that was on sale in his store. When the salesman offered a second hand phone, actually expensive handset saying that it's a very good deal, I interrupted in the ongoing conversation saying, 'Uncle, instead of buying a second hand phone with only a few basic functions, why don't you consider purchasing a brand new, cheap phone? My mom had always told me that people sell their own phones if one or more functions of the phone stop working.'

He replied, 'I buy at least one new cell phone in a month.' I had heard that some people cannot activate their morning bowel movement without newspaper or magazine or even smoking. This middle-aged man was so deeply addicted to social media that as soon as he felt the pressure, he wanted his handset before him to activate bowel movement. He explained to me further that accidently by mishandling the device, it fell into the pot many times. Addiction has reached to the bathrooms now? I could only sympathise with the man! The day is not far when someone would consult me that he or she is an addict of having shower with a protective hand held over his or her favourite device. In fact, knowing the dangerous reality of gadget addiction, I will even believe this.

The traffic government of my city runs a campaign 'don't drink and drive,' but now, modern society has already learnt to drink and drive, turning their latest addiction to conducting a crime relating to driving while using a cellphone. The word accident alone sends shivers down any of our spines.

My chauffer's wife, in an attempt to keep her husband away from answering a call or dialing while driving, set the lock screen image of their only son's (of age two years) picture with the thought in her mind that maybe he will remember his only son before using the cell phone while driving. However, the poor lady fails to understand the modern devices. There wasn't a need to unlock the phone's screen to dial or receive a call. Bluetooth, voice dialing, and headphones have also added to the comfort, which leads to very bad consequences in future.

Chapter 10

DE-ADDICTION CENTRES

Throughout the globe, there are several de-addiction centres with counselors and psychologists working with people, some as young as 9 years old. These counselors and doctors work with children, and even some adults, by encouraging them to take part in more outdoor activities. The outdoor activities are introduced in an attempt to distract, especially the youngsters, from their smartphones and other gadgets. This technique is quite successful to some extent when people are indulged in those activities, but can resort soon to electronics once the activities are stopped. There are no enduring effects of outdoor activities, as the mind does not register for itself what is wrong and what is right.

Moreover, teaching the centre's members about the harmful effects of staying online is another widely used method. The mentors of these centres believe that through education, many will understand the consequences and might actually voluntarily give up electronics. However, this is hardly the case. Once a person is attached or addicted deeply to a tool, he or she would definitely not want to listen to anything against that tool. Hence, these practises can make them even more furious with the people around them and aggravate the already existing problems. Higher number of people are seen to be anxious due to constant provoking and cribbing to leave electronics.

Many people are motivated to give up their virtual lives, and thereby replace them by their real world. This sort of motivation can be an effective tool to some point. Some people, who are affected deeply by pep talks and have high credibility toward people, tend to be very vulnerable toward motivational strategies, and hence, can be helped substantially. Whilst, on the other hand, very firm and strongheaded people who think they are the sole controllers of their lives cannot have their minds changed by any means. They always seem to do whatever they wish to and have extremely undeflected minds. Not only this, if people even leave using gadgets, they start feeling like they've lost a friend or a lover. Addiction is very strong, which leads them into such a state.

The activities and practises done in these centres have not shown very positive outcomes, and have all proven to be futile in some or the other way. But gadget addiction is a very messy problem and needs urgent de-addiction measures. De-addiction from gadgets is a necessity in this advancing era. A practise must be adopted by each of us, which trains our minds and teaches us from within about the beneficial things meant for us. We need to deviate ourselves from electronic world by totally cancelling the thoughts and cravings we get time to time, and practise more mind-relaxing and stress-relieving activities. Brain should be operated by us and must be taught to distract ourselves from technological gadgets.

Chapter 11

HOW CAN ADDICTION BE CURED?

Only remedy to cure gadget addiction is to rationalise the actual cause of addiction of gadgets, rectify it, and eliminate it. Researchers have discovered that the key to all of our problem lies in stress, fast pace life, and competition. We are rushing in panic, in fear, in race that we have no time to analyse where exactly are we going and weather we really want go get there?

Going back to my previous chapter, I had narrated Mr Sujoy's addiction for game of cards, which became such an acute addiction that in a state of severe stress when his daughter suffered pain due to his craving for the game of cards, he used a gadget yet again to cope up with this his high stress. He again opted for game of cards. If every being on this planet, including Mr Sujoy, was being taught to handle stress, handle anxiety, handle fear, handle pain, maintain inner peace, and calm themselves using appropriate measures, then no one will ever resort to using gadgets and everyone will be de-addicted from gadgets. Effective training and developing of mind, body, and soul can be done through simple physical and mental activities, and through watching and controlling one's breathing movements in an integrated practise called 'yoga.'

Everyone must understand that a few minutes spent on improving your mind and body is much more beneficial than wasting hours and hours on destructive tools. Whilst noticing my own technological usage, I realised the influence of my practise of yoga on my online behavioural issues. Yoga has always been a significant part of my life and has helped me to almost totally eradicate the consumption of electronic devices. Not only this, it has played a major role in minimizing the effects of daily usage of some technical gadgets. Through this calming practise, de-addiction can be extremely easy and very helpful in the long run. Yoga is one of the most relaxing and stress-relieving practises, which has no possible drawbacks and can help any human being to improve both mind and body.

Yoga is a very effective practise to solve the problem of addiction by training and developing the mind, body, and soul to be moderate and in a normal state in order to avoid conflicting thoughts between the urge to use gadgets and totally neglect them. Our awareness of our bodies and minds and our inner self is not as sharply developed as it is about the electronic gadgets we are so conveniently equipped with. For example, we do not devote much thought and time to how we sit or stand, how we breathe, how our hearts beat, how our minds function. Our minds are engulfed in technology, and hence, our actions are generally a direct and automatic response to these modern evil devices. As our actions aren't kept in control, we experience some disharmony in the working of our mind and body that we gradually realise the need to attend to ourselves and detach completely from electronics.

Soon, we start to analyse our reactions and search for an understanding of the working of our minds and bodies by doing yoga. In turn, we look for new and better ways to reform our actions. We need to direct our attention within and gain control over ourselves. We have to learn to use our body in such a manner, so as to achieve greater control over the whole organism, physical, mental, and spiritual.

Throughout the globe, there are millions of gadget addicts, but not all of them are aware about using yoga as an activity to de-addict from this dangerous phenomenon. Only a handful of people have used yoga as part of their journey in recovery programs from serious gadget addiction issues to a new life of well-being and emotional stability. As for me, neither did I realise that I have been overusing my iPhone for texting and calling, and my laptop for watching movies and doing Facebook nor did I feel the need to limit my usage. Even after constant pressure from the entire family, I never gave up my electronic devices and kept convincing myself about their worth and utility in my life. Soon, I started yoga as a physical exercise without understanding the deeper implications of yoga in my life. As for me, due to my overdependence on gadgets, I battled to find stability and balance.

Through yoga, there were numerous changes in me, which I never realised, but my friends and close family members noticed those changes and told me about those frequently. Earlier, I used to be detached from normal life and was always dug up in my phone and preferred virtual communication than actually meeting my friends face to face. However, because of consistently practicing yoga, I gained a positive spark in me, and I am motivated ever since to be cheerful and happy around people. Not only this, my irritability also decreased greatly after this calming practise. Nowadays, I am less stressed out and more stable and balanced than ever before.

Whenever I do yoga, I relax with my own thoughts and feel more empowered, more spiritually sound. Whilst practicing yoga, I get a grip on my life, an inner strength that allows me to think for myself, what is wrong, and what is right for me. Accordingly, I am able to set my own targets and limitations in life. I decide for myself that I need to control and keep a check on my growing urge of repeatedly checking phone for updates.

Yoga is a self-enforced activity in which I am left with my own mind to see and understand what is actually happening around me. In all the other de-addicting activities, another mentor or a professional drills in your minds what is good for us and what is not, but the best method is one in which you self-realise everything rather than needing someone else to tell you what you should be doing. In yoga, you are your own god and have to take your own actions instead of depending on someone else.

According to Patanjali's *Yoga Sutras*(a collection of the materials of yoga from older traditions), in the second sutra, the Sanskrit phrase states, 'Yogas citta vrtti nirodha.' This phrase literally translates to 'yoga is restraining the mind stuff (cittas) from taking various forms (vrittis).' This means that through yogic practises and activities, we learn to restrain and control our mind. Once we train our minds and bodies, it avoids taking up any activity, which we do not want it to take. So when we tell and train our minds that we have to control our urge for gadgets and need to reduce our dependence, our mind restrains any activity, which go against our control and our training of the mind. Yoga has cured various types of cancers, so it can easily be used as a tool to detach the mind from the technological world.

Through a highly complex training program, the nervous system can be strengthened, and all the voluntary and major involuntary functions of the body can be brought under direct control of the will. Such a unique achievement in physical culture is only possible the scientific techniques of yoga. All the components of yoga, whether they benefit the mind or the body or the soul, very effectively blend and collaborate to work on specific attributes or causes of addiction in order to eradicate them completely and make one forget about the E-world.

Chapter 12
YOGA CHANGED LIVES

'When people use different things or take substances, they're seeking a certain experience, whether it's escapist or transcendental or just wanting a different psychological state, to get away from whatever is making them unhappy,' explains Sat Bir Khalsa, director of the Kundalini Research Institute, and an assistant professor at Harvard Medical School.

Whenever people are suffering from extreme levels of depression or sorrow, they tend to resort to using excessive amounts of electronic equipment to distract them temporarily from their despondency, and make them feel happier about their lives. However, this method opted is definitely not advisable, as it can have serious consequences such as gadget addiction and social destruction. Hence, to avoid gadget addiction, depression must be combated in the beginning itself.

I know someone who lives in Raipur, Chhattisgarh who embodies the perfect case for depression and it's treatment. She puts up the strongest front in the world. Despite the fact that she is unemployed and depends on her husband for a living, she knows how to fake a smile perfectly. However, despite the cheery, trouble-free façade she presents to the world, she suffers from grave depression. She's been suffering since she used to be a teenager. She would stay in bed until dusk unable to move, to speak, and even to think properly, sobbing at random intervals became a routine activity for her. Sometimes, her depression would take the form of anger, not sadness. She cannot control her emotions; she gets in fight with random people whilst walking down the street, and shouts at everyone she sees in order to take down her fury. She is a loner with absolutely no friends and family due to her short-tempered attitude.

During her college years also, she blew all of the career opportunities provided to her. She used to be too depressed to properly evaluate. She found herself spending hours on the couch, watching television to escape the bad mood and the depressive thoughts evolving in her mind. Also, she started using Facebook and met some strangers online. She became friends with people who hardly knew anything about her life and her habits. She presumes for her happy, virtual world to be her real world. She was engrossed in her iPad all day long. She started forgetting about her real life responsibilities like preparing lunch, arranging the cupboards, and setting the bed sheets. Her husband soon got fed up of her and filed a divorce against her within the next two months. Her situation of depression worsened and needed immediate action. Her technological usage increased even more with her world revolving around Facebook and Twitter. As she had no friends, she constantly checked any and every online gossip of the town, and tried to connect with every person she could find online. She had become crazy for her laptop and iPad. In order to fight her addiction from electronic gadgets, she needed to be happier and more satisfied in her original life. Virtually, she was happier and felt better, but in reality, she was miserable and needed help.

My mother suggested to her about trying out yoga to have a stable mind and be balanced from within. Yoga healed her completely and helped her to regain her cheer, thereby avoiding the need for her to connect with technological gadgets. She started to see and feel concrete, sustained shifts in her mental patterns, emotions, and internal state of being after she began practicing yoga. Yoga uses unique mind-body approach to reduce stress, treat depression, and to enhance overall well-being.

The first step toward removing depressing thoughts from her system was to realise that happiness was her true nature. Just like each one of us, even she has a source of inner bliss, which she might have ignored all her life. However, through yoga, she tapped this inner joy by creating an inner connection with her own inner self. This gives a positive approach to her life. It makes her aware of her inner thoughts, conditions, and desires. She used to constantly be aware of negative and depressing thoughts, but overcame that by asserting her real nature, which was full of bliss. She was also coerced to believe that each one of us is God's child, and he will never want us to be upset or unhappy about anything in life. He, who is the creator of this universe, has blessed us with this life and always has a great future planned for us. This entire world, land and money, everything belongs to him, and he shares all of those resources with us. With this belief in mind, she got positivity in her life and which helped her erase depressive thoughts from her mind.

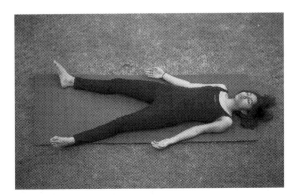

Savāsana(corpse pose):
-Lie down supine
-relax all parts-allow body to 'let go' to gravity.
-break up tension from legs, feet, neck, arms, hands,
*   palms.*
-breathe normally
-do this for 8-10 minutes

Not only this, she started doing yogic meditation (*dharana*) to train her mind and realise for herself. Self-inquiry was paramount. She caught hold of all those mental patterns that unconsciously put her in depressive and negative mood. She shook herself out of these patterns. She tried to live in the present moment and gave the mind a pleasant and positive distraction. Unless she, for herself, did try and was willing to consciously come out of depression, she could actually succeed in overcoming that problem. Self-realisation and self-introspection of her own mind and her thoughts was a necessity to accept the problem and then work on it. Many yogic postures (*āsanas*) can also be beneficial in overcoming depression.

Firstly, she practised the surya namaskara (sun salutation) early morning every day without fail. This is a very good exercise and helped her to remove stress and depression. This sun salutation consists of twelve poses (āsanas) done in a fixed sequence. It gave flexibility to her body and increased the flow of oxygen in her body. It got the adrenaline flowing and relieved depression completely. The adrenaline, which is released from the adrenal glands mentally and physically, prepares the body for any emotion; and in her case, she experienced the feeling of joy due to this adrenaline flow. Her heart rate and breathing rate also became more acute improving, and contributing to her body's positive response. When the sun salutation was done slowly with coordinated breathing movements, it created a feeling of well-being and happiness. Not only this exercise, she also did the *savāsana* (corpse pose) in which she just relaxed with both palms and feet open. Through this pose, she gained entire control of herself, and allowed only the positive thoughts to seep in her brain. Lastly, she even practised *parvatāsana* (mountain pose), which removes any depression felt in mind if this pose is held for two minutes or more.

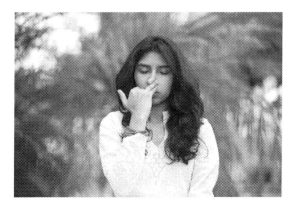

Anuloma Vilomna Pranayama
-Sit in a comfortable meditative posture and use thumb
   and two last fingers for breathing.
-firstly, block the left nostril and with a count of two,
   breathe through the right nostril.
-hold the breath for five seconds and then exhale with
   the count of two though the left nostril.
-now, repeat the same process with inhaling through the
   left nostril and exhaling through the right nostril.

Yogic *pranayama* (breathing exercises) also contribute significantly to reducing depression and anxiety. All the *pranayama* techniques help in removing mind blocks, and improves the circulation of positive energy in body. *Anuloma Vilomna pranayama* (alternate nostril breathing) cleans the energy channels, ensuring that energy flows through the entire body, spreading positive vibes everywhere. Moreover, *bhramari pranayama* (Humming the *M* sound) acts as a calming device creating peace and tranquility within. She observed considerable changes in her attitude, and her perspective toward life after practicing these *pranayamas*.

She was also motivated by her yoga guru to replace issues and depressive behaviour with sane thoughts. This gave her sanity. Due to this, she gained faith in herself, and a new ray of hope of having a better life. She listed down all the negative influences and thoughts on the left side of a piece of paper, and all the positive ones on the right side of the paper. Following this, she let her mind decide for itself which activities, thoughts, and influences will actually benefit her and which will disrupt her well-being. She realised that the saddening things didn't even matter and were actually bullshit'. Through yoga, her mind became very strong and started taking correct decisions for her betterment without her even needing to realise the decisions and outcomes of her contemplation.

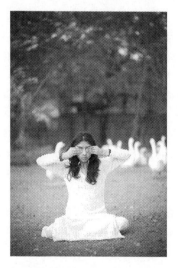

Bhramari pranayama:
-Sit up straight with your eyes closed. Keep a soothed look on your face.
-Place your thumb on the cartilage of your ear and all the four fingers covering your face, primarily eyes.
-taking a deep breath, keep pressing your cartilage in and out as you produce a humming sound through your mouth.
-make a high pitch sound for better results.

After days of rigorous routinal yoga, the yogic practises cured her deeply and helped her to avoid loss and grief. Yoga made her happy and gave her an immense amount of pleasure from within. This mind-body connection calmed her stress response system and contributed to a state of calm. Now, she feels happier and full of energy. She considers herself as living a new life, living away from all the negative people and their negative energies. There is nothing of any sort that upsets her or bothers her anymore. In fact, she is even working with one of the biggest accounting firms of India. She has gained a confidence in herself, her abilities, and does not believe in any materialistic happiness, but in what comes from within. Her reliance on gadgets has reduced to a minimal level. She doesn't feel like using any of the social networking sites and applications like Facebook and Whatsapp to make new friends, and be engrossed in fake, virtual world. No sort of interaction is her source of pleasure anymore. She doesn't use her phone to be updated about the external world or make new friends. She hardly uses her phone for any purpose. She has made her rapport with her real friends even stronger and spends as much quality time as possible with them.

Treating depression through yoga gave her a new life, and a reason to live her life to the fullest. Her overdependence or overusage of laptop and mobile phone, which lead her to being a gadget addict or gadget freak, was also resolved through yoga. Once she came out of her grave depression, she didn't need any of these extrinsic factors to make her happy.

Chapter 13

YOGA AND FORGIVENESS

For most of us, social applications like Facebook and Whatsapp act as a therapy to overcome betrayal. Pretending to have perfect lives even after having imperfect friendships and peer groups is pretty normal for any teenager in this generation. We like to show to the world that our lives are on top of the world, and we don't really need any fake friends to make us happy and satisfied. As we break friendships with our loved ones, which is one of the most fragile relationships in the world, we try to connect with our phones and apps to forget about the broken bond, and try to be best friends with these gadgets. We feel incomplete and lost from within, still not able to accept the fact that we've lost a very dear friend. That loss, which isn't realised by us, affects us in many ways; one of them being, making us a tech-addict. The day we learn to let go of our friendships, and start accepting the fact that we can make our lives much better than before.

A few years back, I read a story online about a teenager named Lauren. Lauren was a 16-year-old girl, same age as me, who went through a very difficult time in her high school due to her friendship issues with her best friend, Paloma. In the summer of 2009, she had a falling out with Paloma, someone she'd known forever. Paloma said some pretty hurtful things to Lauren, and Lauren vowed never to speak to or see her again. And she didn't—for years. Well, at least not directly. However, since Lauren had known Paloma for more than eight years, and had been her best friend for six years, she obviously couldn't let go of her easily and couldn't take her out of her mind. Paloma had formed a permanent residence in Lauren's mind, and no matter how hard she tried, Paloma didn't leave.

Lauren started waking up each morning reliving the conversation the two girls had. She went to bed inventing the conversation they should have had to make amends in their friendship, and during the day, the memory of Paloma's words knotted Lauren's stomach and ruined her appetite. She talked about it to her family, her other friends, pretty much anyone who'd listen. And the more she talked, the hotter the flame of her outrage became. Of course, she focused solely on Paloma's role as the perpetrator and her own role as the aggrieved, never even entertaining the thought that her actions may have contributed a tiny little bit to the problem.

Lauren wanted to feel like everything was normal in her life. She didn't want to cut off from other people and loose them too, creating a huge social mess. She soon reverted to using social networking sites to portray to the exterior world that her life was perfect. She wanted all her online contacts to believe that she was still socially active and wasn't affected by her broken friendship with Paloma. Lauren wanted everyone to believe that everything is normal in her life. She hid her real life behind the screens, and allowed others to judge her on the basis of what she wanted them to think through social applications' profiles. She tried to show herself like an outgoing socialite who loves to hang out with new people and meet more people. Soon, she started using her online world to escape the reality and denied accepting the reality. It became a medium for her to not realise that an important person was missing from her life.

Whilst she was extremely busy faking her not so perfect life, she could not free herself from the shackles of Paloma's friendship, which still existed in the back of her mind. Instead of accepting and letting go of the mishappening that took place, she plunged in further by posting non-stop on different websites.

However, all her efforts were futile. Neither was she able to show Paloma and everyone else how happy she was nor was so much of applications usage helping her in any way. She was being obsessed with showing people false things, especially Paloma, that she wasn't affected by her at all.

Soon, Lauren started forgetting all other activities and concentrated only on putting the best possible façade on her online profiles. It was as if Internet held her captive and captivated her attention completely. To free herself from this weird addiction of posting too much on the Internet, she had to control her mind and let go of Paloma because of whom she was actually turning like this. She started with yoga with the pursuit of physical fitness and relaxing her mind, but didn't really know how it actually helped her move past old hurts that derailed her to a lot of extent due to simple practises of reflecting upon herself and letting go of the past experiences. She tried to practise yoga with internal diatribe in her mind, which never worked too well, compelling her to practise yoga with a free-spirited mind. Hence, she parked her troubles at the door, allowing her body and her mind to breathe a collective sigh of relief, grateful for the ninety-minute respites. It took her several years to learn how to use the principles of yoga to relieve the hurt she felt, and to forgive both Paloma and herself.

Of course, it was impossible for Lauren to forgive Paloma and to condone her behaviour, but she had to let go of the hold Paloma had on her to lead her to a greater freedom and peace of heart. For this to be achieved, she had to forgive Paloma, but not forget about her past actions. She had to learn to honour her feelings and create proper boundaries for herself. Stuffing down the hurt or anger only makes things worse. When Lauren vowed not to think about her pain, she was letting go of it superficially from your mind, but in reality, she was pushing it deeper into her body and heart, both of which constrict around the hurt. To relieve from her heart, she was expressing her disappointments and sorrows through social networking websites. Withholding forgiveness goes against the first and the foremost yoga commandment, *Ahimsa* (non-violence). This not only means that Lauren shouldn't harm her oppressor, Paloma, no matter how aggrieved she felt, it also means that Lauren shouldn't be hurting herself. She was letting the pain go deeper by the over utilization of online websites. This way, she was psychologically harming and ruining herself. Getting stuck in Paloma's transgression made Lauren an anxious mess, coercing her to turn to yogic path from asana and meditation to self-reflection and faith to find forgiveness and move beyond the past.

As renowned *Iyengar* teacher, Patricia Walden explains, 'Our issues are in our tissues.' The inability of Lauren to forgive Paloma definitely manifested as physical contradictions. The pain that Lauren was feeling was lodging almost anywhere in the heart, diaphragm, or belly. By focusing on the breath while practicing *asanas*, Lauren noticed that she was holding on to a kind of pain. And by releasing tension in her muscles, she could let go of that discomfort. Poses like *matsyāsana* allow breath to flow unrestricted and can open up the heart. This heart opening effect made Lauren feel nurtured and loved, relieving her anger, and curing her super anxious mode.

This further led to a complete decline in her online updating activities. Lauren was in complete control of her transient emotions, which led her to being fake on social sites. While on mat, she could almost immediately feel how her emotions affected her body. She used to forget to breathe whenever her anger for Paloma resurfaced, and her body used to stiffen up whenever she got frustrated.

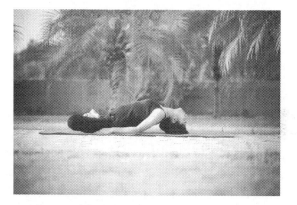

Matsyasāna(the fish pose):
- Assume padmasana- the foot-lock in a manner that the feet are set against the respective opposite groins, with soles turned upward.
- taking aid of arms, throw weight of trunk on elbows one after the other and, with inhalation, lean back gradually and lie down flat.
- fold arms above head.
- maintain the pose for 6 seconds and return to starting position of padmasana with exhalation.

After initial *asana* practise, Lauren began with meditation. Meditation opened up new doors for Lauren, which she never imagined would ever open up. She started practicing *metta bhavana* (loving-kindness meditation). This form of meditation got feelings of compassion into Lauren who soon completely compromised on her part, and even ended up becoming better best friends than ever with Paloma due to her low level of short temper this time. When she started off with this meditation technique, she would meditate and then become accepting Paloma as the traitor all over again. She would forgive Paloma, but would never consider herself as the perpetrator too. However, she never stopped meditation, and much to her surprise, her resentment toward Paloma faded.

Lauren was encouraged by yoga teacher to firstly get clear on what her story was—exactly what she felt—so that it would conceptualise what happened and then to drop it. Retelling and recalling the incidents made no sense. Hence, she focused more on her feelings of the story rather than the story itself. Remembering the story could have only led to justification of those feelings, not forgiving. When Lauren caught hold of her thoughts regarding the incidents with Paloma, she only reviewed her feelings and the effects the fight had on her specifically. She realised that Paloma, who she thought was the traitor, could manage everything and not be affected by anything, whilst she was the one who was using all the power and contacts she had to show to her ex-best friend how perfect her life was without Paloma. Lauren thought that the only solution to her temper was to forgive Paloma and become friends with her again.

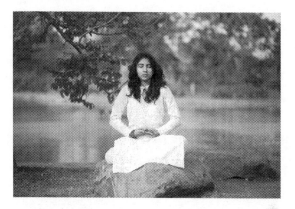

Metta Bhavana:
-Sit in a comfortable posture preferably sukhasana
   or padmasana with both your hands just below
   your naval.
-try to sit with full concentration and focus.
-now, start thinking positive things about yourself and
   the people and things around you.
-try to eradicate negativity completely from your
   system and only think about friendly thoughts.
-This practise will make your attitude toward life and
   people very positive.

Gradually, Lauren learned to forgive; and during her meditation practise, she completely let go of her anger toward Paloma. Once she felt better from within, she called up Paloma and asked if they could meet and talk over a cup of coffee. Both of them had dealt with the situation smartly resorting to becoming great friends again. Due to this, Lauren's obsession of utilising too many social networking sites also reduced to a minimal level. She just didn't feel like using any of these damaging technological devices, as she became extremely busy mending things with Paloma.

Chapter 14

DEVELOPING PRACTISE AND DETACHMENT

Yoga sutra, which is a compilation of the basic yogic fundamental, states in the sutra 1.12, *Abhyasavairagyabhyam tannirodha*, that to achieve a certain state of yoga, we need to develop practise and detachment. Through this, we can gain stability of body and mind, and strengthen our power of will and determination. Once we're determined to achieve something and know how to have a strong will to reject the utilisation of gadgets, we can disconnect our lives from the influence of these foul devices. To be successful in our endeavor of de-addiction, we need to methodically practise (*abhyasa*) and detach (*vairagya*).

Persistent practise of detachment from gadgets enables us to concentrate on other vital things in life, and replace the importance of gadgets with more fruitful activities. The reflective discipline of detachment from technology helps us to avoid the charms and temptations of the addictive E-world. Detachment or non-attachment builds an internal strength in us to discard the electronic devices that are unpleasant, useless, and undesirable, and to limit our usage when we do need to use them for some petty works. Through detachment, we become productive and perform our actions skillfully whilst totally neglecting our phones, laptops, etc.

A few years back, in around 2012, I knew someone who was crazy over Indian cricket. He wouldn't miss a single match in the Indian premiere league. He was a huge fan of the captain of Chennai Super Kings, Mahendra Singh Dhoni. In 2012 summer, Chennai Super kings (CSK) was winning almost every match. His home was struck by CSK fever with all his family members, especially him, hooked to the television. He became passionately involved with the matches, and found himself staying up late watching various replays against different teams online, sometimes until 3 a.m.! Before long, he began to notice the unfortunate effects of his enthusiasm. Because he'd wake up groggy in the morning, he'd end up skimping on his classes and would feel short-tempered throughout the day. Once he realised that his burgeoning obsession with Chennai Super Kings replays and players was compromising his mood and his ability to be focused and present, he gratefully reaffirmed his commitment to practise of neglecting the television programmes, and his goal of a more focused, present, and easeful state of being. Following this, he was able to limit his late nights on computer. He was advised by his school counselor to follow the yogic techniques of practise (*abhyasa*) and detachment (*vairagya*), which helped him de-addict himself from his television fever.

Patanjali who is considered one of the pioneers of yoga, and the author of the sacred *Yoga Sutra*, said, 'Practise and detachment are two of the very first tools to help us in this process of refining the mind toward clear perception and deeper connection with the self.' My brother followed his footsteps very wisely and concentrated on devoting himself toward practise and detachment. He practised all the activities, which helped him quiet his mind, made him forget about his cricket matches, and focused his attention out of the television world and in the real world. He started running and cycling regularly with my father. Both of these physical activities calmed his mind and deviated his attention away from cricket. Slowly and eventually, my brother started turning out to be a high-level long distance runner with his growing inclination toward running. He started taking running extremely seriously and started representing our school in many inter-school competitions.

Other than practicing running, which became his passion, my brother even let go of habits and tendencies, which impeded in his well-being. It was a very difficult thing for him to do, but it was best for his health and his running to let go of laptop to watch replays and television to watch live matches. He really needed to de-addict himself from these visual devices to retain his good health and mind. Eventually, He learnt to let go of his habits of watching late night cricket to run early morning. He understood that to practise his running regularly, he will have to give up his cricket matches. This realisation was the first step toward his detachment with watching cricket. In his sessions with his school counselor, he was only counseled to leave those activities, which impeded in his progress. He did not give up going to lunches and dinners with his friends circle, or going out for picnics with our grandparents every fourth Sunday of the month, but only gave up his late night matches, which affected his early morning running activity.

Abhyasa (practise) and *vairagyam* (detachment) are like two sides of the same coin. The first is moving toward the goal and practicing our endeavours, the second is clearing our paths of obstacles. The important thing about detachment is that when we are strongly and positively focused on our goals, giving up what's getting in our way will, ideally, not feel like an enormous struggle. The more dedicated we become to our early morning practises, the more we can see the positive changes that happen in our lives as a result of that strong dedication and the easier it will become to forgo staying up late to surf the Internet; and in my brother's case, look for more matches.

Also, simple visualization with the inhalation and exhalation of breath is helpful for cultivation of that, which supports us, and letting go of that which does not. In a comfortable posture with eyes shut, a few conscious, relaxed breaths must be taken. A simple visualization must be done during inhalation. During inhalation, whatever is supportive of our goals must be practised with strength and confidence. Only positive thoughts related to our aspirations must seep in. Whilst during exhalation, we must let go of any destructive activities, which do not support us. Our decisions of minimizing the usage and dependence on technology must be soaked into our brains and effectively implemented during exhalation.

Not only should we let go of materialistic things like gadgets, but also intangible things like fear, doubt, and negative thinking. Whilst inhalation, we must practise steps, which lead us to fulfill our ambitions; and during exhalation, we must decide to replace the utility of gadgets with much more desirable objects.

The great yoga guru, Sadhguru, also speaks about addiction and has said, 'If they did not think it is better than whatever else is available around, they would not do it. In their perspective, it is good.' His scholarly words help us understand that in order to let go of our addictions, we need to find something better as a replacement. We cannot just give up our phones or laptops because we've been asked to do so, or we've been deviated by Sunday school or something better. A certain inclination, seriousness, and a level of practise must be there for any activity, which we do to replace the utility of gadgets. However, in the long run, those activities such as swimming or knitting should no longer be a distraction but a passion. From being addicted to gadgets, we must learn to be addicted to our passions and must have the inbuilt desires to fulfill our passions.

Following our dreams and fulfilling our aspirations and passions does not cost anything, neither does health nor money. Unless we do not practise activities or hobbies of our interests, we absolutely cannot detach ourselves from these technological devices.

'Behind any accomplishment, there is always a force, desire.' The level or the intensity of detachment depends on desire for practise (*abhyasa*). Victory over any activity and control over mind is only possible for those of us with intense desire. In intense desire, also, there are three stages or classes: mild, intermediate, or supreme. A burning desire to attain mastery over mind and over our passions is the first—and most essential—attribute to de-adddict ourselves from technology. The strength of the desire determines how easy it is for us to forget about the evil devices. If we have a mild desire to do something, we lack motivation and the drive to achieve something. Our inclination toward a certain level of practise is very low. We can easily extinguish this desire by the fear of failure. The spark in us is too small to propel us forward. With this kind of desire, we know the value of achieving the higher goal of life; we wish to attain it, but do not have enough motivation to really start. We enjoy daydreaming and lack practise. With this lack of practise, it can be extremely rigorous, and a long process for us to de-addict ourselves. With intermediate desire, we are endowed with a higher degree of intense desire, but still not that powerful enough to carry us through. We might be overly zealous about our desire to attain our goals, but when confronted with obstacles later, we decide to drop our desires. Having this desire does help in distracting us from electronics till some extent, as it is very difficult to neglect them in the long run. With supreme desire, the desire is so strong that it consumes all other desires. The desire to achieve something overpowers the desire to use gadgets. With our strong desires in mind, we are motivated to settle for nothing but our goals. The intensity of desire is important because it determines how easy and quick will it be for us to de-addict ourselves permanently from technology.

Chapter 15

ANXIETY VS *AHIMSA* (NON-VIOLENCE)

Being anxious about things has never done any good to anyone. We're all anxious about different things and aspire to have different things in life. Our anxiety levels shoot up before petty events and for small things. If we don't get what we want, then our overanxious minds start thinking negatively about different people and different things. That negative thinking, which is evoked in us, is known as violence. This does not only refer to physical violence, but also refers to the mental pain we cause to each other, and negative thoughts we have about other people. When we practise *ahimsa* (non-violence), which is one of the moral restraints, we swear to love each other and not think ill about our own people. In this cut throat world, not even one of us is innocent. Each one of us covets a perfect life, and more than that, better than our friends and relatives. We have an inbuilt need to prove to them how perfect we are, and how our social status is the best among everyone. By practicing *ahimsa,* we subdue the negative thoughts toward others in us.

One form of anxiety, which all of us teenagers go through, is Social Anxiety Disorder. In this, we become social climbing desperate people who have a paralysing fear of being judged by other people or embarrassing ourselves in a public setting.

We go to great lengths to limit any and every interaction with others, perhaps even eschewing opportunities to make friends or business contacts, or go out for socializing. This is just not simple shyness. Those of us with this kind of disorder cannot simply 'get over' our discomfort, thereby, getting forced into a public situation, or one where we have to interact with another individual, can be traumatizing and debilitating for us. Many of us can also start panicking weeks before we are due to meet with another person, or if at all, we believe sometimes that we are being judged or watched by others in a large setting. When we suffer this kind of an anxiety, we try to make virtual contacts and make attempts to gain fame on the Internet. The overanxious state of our minds makes us turn to extreme gadget usage to cope with the stress, especially if we encounter an influential personality and embarrass ourselves in front of him/her.

Moreover, the negativity toward other people blocks the flow of positive energy in us, leaving with excessive amounts of negative energy. This excessive negativity flows around in our body, and slowly, we make an attempt to consume this from of energy; we utilise this energy by distracting our minds and thinking about video games and other forms of online entertainment. This overusage of negative vibes and energy clutters our minds and increases our overdependence on E-devices significantly!

The main reason why we suffer from this kind of an anxiety is low self-esteem and negativity toward other people. The day we get rid of that negative attitude toward people, that day we can communicate with real people rather than faceless ones on the Internet and increase the efficiency of our brain by not using too many technological gadgets. We are always scared of people and think of them as monsters, but in reality, when we correct this attitude of ours, half the things can be mended. We always get bad thoughts and negative vibes from people around us, which don't even exist in reality, but they do in the back of our minds. Practising *Ahimsa,* which refers to eradicating negative feelings from our system toward ourselves and others, can help us significantly to remove the fear of other people. Following this practise, we can get back to the real life, meet more new faces, and not be hooked to virtual life just by engraving in our psyche that everyone surrounding us is good, and we do not have to be afraid of anyone.

It is extremely important to remove all sorts of negativity from our minds to get outside in the real world. We will have to relinquish hostility and irritability, and instead, make space within our consciousness for peace. In that space, we must resolve all the anger, separation, and aggression. This will let others be who they are and also allow us to relate to the world in a whole new way. Mahatria Rā once said that the most important aspect of blocking negativity from our minds is to stop thinking 'I am holier than thou.' The day our ego mind stops operating and thinking that I am more superior than the other person, that day we can let go of the negative attitude toward people. Various yogic practises can also help us reflect upon the negativity in our minds, thereby incorporating *ahimsa* in our lives.

Yoga allows us to calmly transform ourselves without being acted out in the world. While doing various *asanas,* when we perform the poses gracefully without force, we develop calmness from within. Our mind becomes more stable and we start gaining feelings of compassion for people. Patanjali defines *asana* as '*sthira sukham asanam*'. He says that whenever we do any *asanas,* we must try to make an effort to reach the maximum capacity, but also know our limits and mustn't harm ourselves in the process of performing an *asana*. The *asana*, which we practise, must be steady or firm and comfortable. *Asanas* like *virbhadrasana I* (warrior pose) give us an excellent stretch in the back of the knee relieving the stress hormones to a greater extent and making us feel positive about everyone around us.

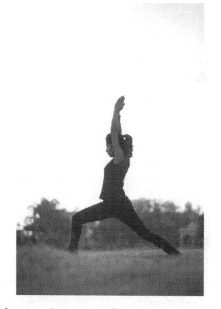

Virbhadrasāna 1(warrior pose):
- Stand straight in tadasana. While breathing out, move your feet so that they are at around at a distance of 4 feet from each other. Raise your arms so that they are perpendicular to the ground and parallel to each other.
- point your right foot outwards towards the right side.
- twisting your lower abdomen, shift your turn your body toward the right side.
- fold your right leg outward and join both the hand upwards.

Different meditative mantras can also aid in the recovery to positive thinking. However, we must take precaution and never meditate when nagging thoughts have completely clogged up our minds, and we are unable to stay focused at the object of our meditation. At that time, instead of forcing to stay in meditation, it is best to quit the practise, and go for a peaceful walk to clear the head. Meditation soothes us from within, creating positive vibes for people around us. Whilst practicing various different kinds of *pranayama* (breathing exercises), especially those involving retention of breath, we mustn't be tempted to hold the breath beyond our capacity. This might severely strain our system and can cause more harm than desired benefits. When we do comfortable breathing exercises, we experience a sense of satisfaction from inside, which generates a very friendly energy in us, driving us to interact and know more happy and similar faces.

Yoga is a very effective tool, which can cure the social anxiety disorder. These small steps can be really helpful in building up self-confidence, which we require to communicate with strangers and well known personalities. Once we can confidently and smartly meet more people, we can detach ourselves from the faceless people on Internet. Our addiction to Internet and technological devices can be decreased to a greater extent as soon as we step in the real world.

Chapter 16

CONTROLLING POWER OF *ĀSANAS*

In this advancing era, video games have become every teenager's best friends. In the year 2000, Mrs Woolley's son, Shawn, became addicted to an online video game called Everquest. Within three months, he quit his school, detached himself from all his friends and family, and was up all night playing. Despite Mrs Woolley's efforts to help him get his life back together, he committed suicide only a year and a half after being introduced to the game.

Shortly after Shawn's suicide, Mrs Woolley did an interview with the *Milwaukee Journal Sentinel*, and that's when she realised how many families are being broken up and suffering like hers. She wanted to warn as many people as possible that these games can take control of their lives just like drugs or alcohol. Some gamers told her one can become addicted in less than twenty-four hours. Once a gamer has gone from social gaming to addicted gaming, he can't go back. Whenever someone consulted her about this issue, she always shared the same notion, 'Games can be a drug of choice and need to be looked at that way.'

Gaming addiction is a sort of gadget addiction, which has the same disastrous effects as compared to alcohol or drugs addiction. Demographically, any age group can be trapped in the shackles of addictive video games. Many colleges recognise that video games cause a huge percentage dropout, some colleges have even hired some counselors to deal with excessive gaming. No college throughout the globe is willing to waste a scholarship on a gamer; hence, in the interview itself, they've started asking students if they've got even a little inclination toward video games. Not only college-going students, high schoolers are no less. Many high school teenagers are wasting their brilliant mind power by spending too much time and energy on these virtual games. Grown married women tend to play social games like Farmville, SIMS, and Second Life. They all end up leaving their families and husband and leaving their children behind. Grown men leave their homes and spend all their resources in playing games.

Mrs Woolley, as mentioned above, has been affected passively by some other addict. Mrs Woolley is not an addict herself, but her son, who was an addict, has had a profound impact on his mother. She was so deeply impacted by the son's activity that she led to awareness amongst others about the harms of gaming addiction. If a passive person can be so affected, it is impossible to imagine also the consequences on the addict himself. Misery and suicide are some of the very few dangers. It is of utmost necessity to stop playing these virtual and spend time in the real life. To find the solution to this gaming, finding out why exactly are we all driven to consume so many virtual video games is very important.

One reason why we all are engrossed in video games is because they give us a sense of worth and accomplishment. Whenever we kill the opponent or reach the end of a level, we become too happy and gain a sense of control. The control, which we probably don't have in real life, we tend to find in virtual life. In the gaming world, we are the supreme leader of ourselves and gain a feeling of independence. Psychologically, any human being craves for joy, for pleasure, for a sense of control, and independence. Video games provide all these needs easily so there is no way a person will ever voluntarily detach himself or herself from these games.

Scientifically, clearing up each level of a video game with ease gives a strong sense of sense satisfaction. This petty accomplishment is experienced as mini reward by our brain, releasing the neurochemical dopamine, and tapping into same neuro-circuitry involved in addiction, reinforcing our actions. Despite its well known reputation of being a pleasure chemical, it also cements our activities and trains us to continue performing them.

Performing and attaining complex *yogāsanās* or yogic postures can also increase the level of happiness in any person. We need to replace the obsession with video games with passion for attaining each and every *āsanās*. Poses like the *chakrasāsanā* or the *bakāsanā* challenge us both physically and mentally. Practising poses like these and being successful in them creates a very positive feeling, and makes us feel much more independent in life.

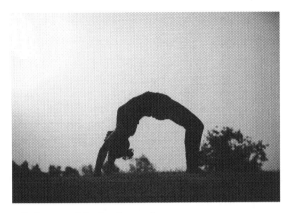

Chakrasana(the bridge pose):
-Lie down on your back with feet apart.
-bend your knees
-bring your palms under the shoulders such that
*   fingers point towards shoulders and elbows are*
*   shoulder width apart.*
-with a gentle inhalation, life your hips up and try to
*   take all the weight on your hands and on your feet.*
-keep inhaling and exhaling normally.

Substituting online game and video games with these postures is not only beneficial for both mind and body, but also gives us the same control as given by *āsanās*. We feel more powerful and in control after staying in these poses for long. Due to them being so difficult, if we become successful in achieving them, we gain confidence in our bodies.

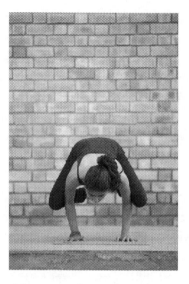

Bakasana(the crow pose):
-Squat on a block or a floor and put your hands
     shoulder distance apart.
- lift the hips higher than the shoulders and look
     forward.
- squeeze the knees outside of the triceps
-pull the navel in and lift up
- breathe very deeply and slowly practise lifting a foot
     at a time, or both feet, off the ground.

Once we get onto the mat and get mastery of any difficult posture, we ooze with self-confidence. Just replacing the hard work of four hours to get the declaration by the computer 'you win' with practising *yogāsanās* only for ten minutes can give you your body's declaration and approval. Your soul from within feels content and satisfied and more powerful than ever. The yoga *āsanās* are a way to feel good without the addictive behaviour attached with video games. Exercise assists the body in boosting the brain's serotonin levels, thus, elevating mood. An elevated mood also aids in boosting confidence, and slowly and gradually helps one to recover totally from video games. Moreover, you start to realise that you are own boss of your mind and body and have to keep a check and control on it. *Āsanās* are one of the most complex physical mechanisms, and gaining mastery over these is one of the biggest achievements according to the human psyche.

Another reason why we are all so allured by the video gaming world is that gives us new opportunities, which we might not get in our daily lives. We get totally addicted to the fantasyland the games take us to. In the year 2008, in Russia, a 17-year-old boy named Egor got addicted to strange cases lighthouse mystery game. He started considering himself a detective and started engrossing his brain totally into that video game. One reason why he was in love with that particular mystery game was the type of situations it offered to him. There were some typical imaginary situations, which he would have never experienced otherwise if he had not started playing this game; for example, solving a puzzle inside a cat's stomach to unlock the house door's lock. His obsession with the game had terrible effects, and soon, by September, he was diagnosed with mental problems and was admitted to a long-term support program. Once, in the middle of the night, he walked back home from the support program, which was almost like five miles away, without notifying anyone or seeking anyone's permission just to finish off the level on which he was stuck. Then at his own elder brother's wedding, the first wedding in the family, he left during the ceremony to play and didn't return for the rest of the day.

Many people noticed that he wasn't at the reception, and later, everyone discovered he had left in the middle of the wedding and walked home to continue playing his game. He would have never have done that before his addiction. He loved parties and socializing.

He needed some urgent help! One of his aunts, when she was visiting his mother during her birthday reunion, told Egor to try yoga. He was already on a very bad stage and had become completely dumb and didn't understand anything. His aunt spoke to his mother, and convinced her to make him join a yoga class nearby. It was impossible for her to send him due to his weakness, but she called home a yoga teacher for him. He was asked to practise only *āsanās* in the early stage to get him out of his addiction. The teacher counseled him in a very video game kind language, and told him about very different *āsanās*, which we wouldn't have thought of or done on a daily basis outside his mat or his yoga class. Soon he started realising that yoga is not only about physical fitness, it's about fun. He could pretend to be a tree in his yoga class (in *vrikshāsanā*). Yoga gave him the excuse to pretend to be a tree even though nothing of that sort ever existed in his daily schedule. It taught him about trying new and weird things without fear. He tried many weird *āsanās*, which he wouldn't have thought of early on and started deriving fun out of them.

Slowly and gradually, he stopped playing that mystery game completely and instilled the technique of *āsanās* in his daily practise.

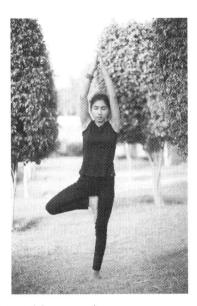

Vrikshāsanā(the tree pose)-
-Stand tall and straight with arms by the side of your body
-bend your right knee and place the right foot high up on your left thigh. The sole of the foot should be places flat and firmly near the root of the thigh.
-make sure that your left leg is straight. Try to balance in this.
-once you are steadily balanced, look straight in front of you. Your body should be like a stretched elastic band.
-with slow exhalation, gently bring down your hands from sides and gently release the right leg.
-now, repeat the same process with the opposite leg.

Āsanās are a very important aspect of yoga, and can be really helpful in elevating an individual's self-esteem and making them experience new and unordinary things

Chapter 17
INCULCATING *APARIGRAHA*

One of the primary reasons why we are overdependent on gadgets and tend to overuse them is the excess of technological devices we own. Reducing the quantity of the devices we own can be one of the simplest solutions for us. If we won't have so many choices to choose from, our consumption will automatically decrease with time. In yoga, there is the practise of *aparigraha*, which means to practise non-possessiveness and non-covertness. It is the decision to not hoard or accumulate any materialistic things through greed, but rather, to develop an attitude of stewardship toward the material world.

Once we get too much stuff into our homes, we need to take care of it and bound to use it. We tend to utilise the things till the very end in an attempt to make the commodity's utility worth its price. In the same process, we become addicted to the commodity. Hence, in this commercial world, *aparigraha* is a must and needs to be practised seriously so that nobody ends up being addicted to technology anymore.

In the *Yoga Sutra* (collection of basic principles of yoga) 2.39, Patanjali states, '*Aparigrahasthairye janma kathanta sambodhah*'. By this sutra, he emphasizes on lack of desire.

He says one should not be greedy to acquire more and more. We must follow simplicity and stability (*sthairye*) and not aim to grasp. For example, if we have one PC at home, we need not have a laptop and an iPad along with it. A mind, which is free from the tension of caring for and using the things often, can see more. The brain, which is given by the God to think and process, does only that and does not get involved in any materialistic electronic devices. Patanjali also explains that our acquisitions are a burden. They come in the way of our freedom and restrict our thinking. They not only demand time and money, but also take away our energy and become a source of worry.

Before buying any new devices into our houses, we need to ask ourselves: Do I need this new device for my role in life? As a parent? As a businessman? As a teacher? Or am I just accumulating stuff out of my own fear and greed? If we do not consider these essential questions, our gadgets can take over. Once this happens, we start being identified with our gadgets because of our attachment with them. It's easy to think that we are our gadgets, but those will come and go. Our personality needs to be strong, so that we are not attached to any gadget so closely and are willing to let go of them easily. We need to constantly get rid of gadgets, which we do not require and are just using unnecessarily from time to time.

Graham Hill is an American who cured his addiction with his electronic devices by following the policy of *aparigraha*. He had a habit of buying everything, and then using everything even if it was not required. He bought everything for namesake, and then used it just to keep himself satisfied. He had a giant house crammed with stuff—electronics and cars and appliances and gadgets. Somehow, this stuff ended up running his life, or a lot of it. The things he consumed ended up consuming him. He said, 'We live in a world of surfeit stuff, of big box stores, and twenty-four-hour online shopping opportunities. Members of every socioeconomic bracket can and do deluge themselves with products. There isn't any indication that any of these things makes anyone any happier. In fact, it seems the reverse may be true.' For him, it took him fifteen years to get rid of all the inessential things he had collected, and he started living a bigger, better, richer life with less.

His gadget addiction began in 1998 in Seattle when he and his partner sold their Internet consultancy company, Siteworks, for more money than they thought they'd earn in a lifetime. To celebrate, Graham bought a four-storey 3,600 square foot turn of the century house in the happening Capitol Hill neighbourhood, a ton of gadgets like Audible. com mobile player, an audiophile-worthy five-disc CD player, and lot of types of computers and earphones. His assistant went to various more appliance and electronic stores, and sent Graham pictures of the stores and things. He shuffled through many pictures and proceeded on a virtual shopping spree. All his acquisitions weren't necessities for him, but he still hadn't realised that. He was trying to use everything, but did not really lead a very happy life. He was alone and spent all his day listening to music or doing something on the internet, mostly surfing the online shopping sites.

Soon, he started wondering why his theoretically upgraded life didn't excite him anymore and made him more anxious than before. His life was becoming unnecessarily complicated. There were devices to be plugged into their respective charging ports, lawns to mow, and cars to be washed. He was becoming more and more exhausted day passing day. He decided to move to a more calming place. He shifted to a 1,900 square feet apartment, and did not take any of his belongings with him. The first few days were extremely difficult and painful for him, as he had to leave his brand new Nokia phone at the old house along with his music player and his iPads. He felt very lonely and dull without these devices. It was as if his life had turned upside down and become completely monochrome. He had difficult time adjusting without the E-devices, but soon, he realised that he felt content from within. He just wasn't wasting his energy on things he didn't need anymore. He had learnt to live with things, which he actually needed, and surely his technological gadgets weren't one of them.

Chapter 18

BLOGS

Author's blogs published in newspaper.

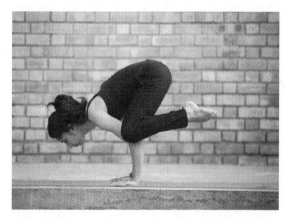

1. Yoga, the Product of Globalisation (*vaishvikaran*)

The world observed the international day of yoga on June 21, and at least 177 countries participated in a thirty-five-minute programme that had been devised for the purpose. A thirty-five-minute yoga day celebration started with a prayer in Sanskrit from the Rig Veda (one of the four vedas which are ancient texts) and end with another.

After mathematics, science, and Ayurveda, yoga is the next marvelous contribution from India to the entire world toward globalisation. The dream of tying the people of the whole world in a common thread was possible through Yoga, which also means addition. If an export could be measured by number of consumers, then Yoga is the most successful business throughout the globe.

From it being free of cost in the very beginning, yoga is now a booming global billion-dollar industry. Corporates have picked it up too and gained media attention for offering yoga classes at workplaces to their employees. Corporate yoga is one of the most common forms of profession nowadays.

Yoga's beneficial effects have been challenged, tested, and verified many times across the world. There have been plenty of evidences due to all the findings that yoga is a contributing factor to the brain gains too.

- Yoga is the fourth fastest growing industry globally.
- There are 300 million people practicing yoga worldwide and 83 per cent of whom are females.
- There are more than fifty yoga styles of which:
  1. Hatha
  2. Ashtanga
  3. Bikram
  4. Vinyasa

are most popular styles.

- Yoga practitioners have 87 per cent less chance of heart diseases.
- Some 73 per cent of practitioners choose yoga for stress management.

2. Shiva is considered as supreme Lord
    (first teacher) of yoga

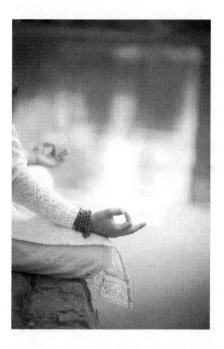

Lord Shiva is considered to be the first teacher of the science of Yoga. Also called *Yogeshwara*, the lord of Yoga, Shiva symbolizes balancing and calming effect of all Yoga practises.

There's a famous story about how yoga originated from Lord Shiva. Lord Shiva danced on the mountains or sat absolutely still. He was either still or dancing madly. Suddenly, all gods in the heaven saw him and felt that something is happening to this guy. He is having such a great time, and we are missing all the fun, so what's the matter? Then they reached out to Lord Shiva to learn the method and Lord Shiva then started teaching various forms of yoga depending upon who he was teaching. The word yoga here did not mean various postures or breathing techniques, but the science of how to take ultimate creation (mankind) to its maximum possibility. These teachings took place near Kedarnath.

The first part of Shiva's teachings were to his own wife, Parvati. The second part was to *Sapta Rishis* or the seven sages who then passed on their knowledge to the rest of mankind. The *Nath Yogis* also, who gave us tantric yoga, hatha yoga, and siddha yoga, were followers of Lord Shiva. Lord Shiva did not give any philosophical instructions, but instead, he just explained some techniques to liberate the soul from the limitations of the body and the mind and experience true blissful state. These techniques got refined over the centuries by various renowned masters who perfected this art, and this is how the wisdom of yoga was passed on through the ages.

Shiva is the master of *asanas*, particularly the seated poses, which are the most important of all the *asanas*. He is usually portrayed in either *Siddhasana* or *Padmasana* (lotus pose), often surrounded by animals that symbolize the other *asanas* as well. Shiva is the great guide to meditation, teaching us to observe, contemplate, and not react. This reality of Shiva is the power of silence and stillness, and works through inaction, peace, and balance in which we are centered in one's own being.

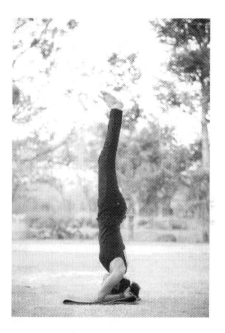

3. You Don't Choose Yoga, Yoga Chooses You

I've grown up hearing from my dad, 'I can't do yoga! My body is stiff' every time my mother forced him to do yoga with her. Every morning, my mom would find different ways of convincing him to accompany her to Sayaji club, Indore for everyday yoga practise. Later, while seeing my parents, I realised that body is never stiff, whilst the mind maybe! It's in our mind when we decide whether we will be able to do yoga or not. Maharishi Patanjali has also rightly said that the fear of going into any yogic practise comes from the mind, not the body. Given a proper guidance, we can attempt every part of yoga.

If ever you decide to measure your ability of practicing yoga, the only thing flashing in your mind will be a person either going into *asanas* or in deep state of meditation. However, seldom do we realise that yoga is much, much more than merely getting into *asanas* or breathing right. Asanas is merely one of the eight limbs (branches) of yoga.

Breath is the first fundamental of life, and it's the only fundamental of yoga. If you can breathe, you can practise yoga. Breathing right with purpose and with awareness can be a solution for almost everything. It isn't just about making your body more flexible and healthy, it's about making your lifestyle more flexible and healthy. Breathing acts as a bridge between your mind and your body. Yoga, in its true sense, is a lifestyle, a culture, a prayer, and lastly, it's the yogic way of living and thinking. It's a practise to feel truly alive. Practicing yoga is saving hours of anxiety, hours of stress, and hours of negativity around.

Some feel beautiful when they look good. Yes, they do! But a yogi feels beautiful while feeling strong, feeling self-loved, feeling a kind of peace of mind. Practising yoga is to feel magnificently intelligent and miraculously happy within. I have realised that social media and zero figure stigma have confused the minds claiming that only lean and flexible bodies should practise yoga, but that notion astutely false. Everybody is fit for yoga, and anyone regardless of weight, age, shape, size, or stamina can benefit from it.

After practising yoga, your body might take weeks to reflect changes, but your mind and thoughts and emotions will notice the changes instantly. The working of internal organs will return to their original capacity and make you feel smooth and light, and there you are, the energy has started to sprout and travel in every part of your body, while making you calm outside. Then understand the sign that you have certainly laid the foundation of becoming a yogi and building a community ahead where everyone who wants to explore personal transformation is welcomed into.

4. We Have Limited Number of Breaths—Breathe Slow and Deep

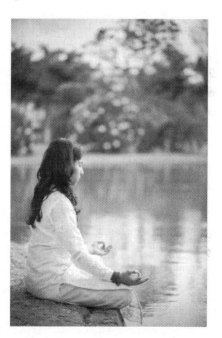

Every time anything used to go wrong, my maa (my paternal grandma) use to blame destiny saying our destiny is drafted at our birth itself. I used to take her approach as a typical orthodox. But the same is said in modern yogic teachings! They say a certain amount (number) of breaths are allotted to us at the time of birth, and if this is true, every slow deep breath will prolong our life; hence, the better we breathe, the better we live. And before we get into the right or wrong breathing techniques, let me tell you; similar to learning to play an instrument, we can train the body to improve its breathing techniques.

A normal person breathes shallow (superficially) about eighteen times a minute, and with each inhalation, he takes in half a litre of air. But a yogi breathes deep and only 12–13 times a minute, but inhales 4 ½ litres of air with each breath. Though the quantity of air reaching the lungs per minute is the same in both the cases, but the quantity of oxygen, which is actually absorbed, and gaseous toxins expelled out in yogi's breathing pattern is more.

In our day-to-day life, it is quite impossible to keep conscious of the breaths all day long and during our daily work. But whenever we remember about breathing deep, we must breathe slowly, deeply, and with awareness, utilising the technique of yogic breathing. One or two minutes of this practise is more beneficial than fifty-nine minutes of shallow breathing and increases our vitality and rejuvenates us.

There's a simple way to check your pattern of breathing. Place your right hand on your chest and your left hand on your abdomen. As you breathe, see which hand rises more. If your right hand rises more, you are a chest breather. If your left hand rises more, you are an abdominal breather. Chest breathing (rapid and shallow) is inefficient because it results in less oxygen transfer to the blood. Whereas abdominal breathing causes more oxygen to flow in blood resulting in improved energy and immunity, and stimulates the sense of relaxation, which is known as the yogic way of breathing and is the base for many breathing exercises.

Let us learn to breath the yogic way:

- Take a slow deep breath in through your nose, imagining that you are sucking in all the air in the room and hold it for a count of seven (or as long as you are able to, not exceeding seven).
- Slowly exhale through your mouth for a count of eight. As all the air is released with relaxation, gently contract your abdominal muscles to completely evacuate the remaining air from the lungs.
- It is important to remember that we deepen respirations not by inhaling more air, but through completely exhaling it. Roughly, exhalation should be twice as long as inhalation.

The yogic breathing becomes even more efficient with the addition of *ujjayi pranayama*, which produces a slight snoring sound. This *ujjayi* breathing is possible in every *asana* as it has an extraordinary revitalizing effect. We can consciously use breathing to regulate blood pressure, heart rate, blood circulation, digestion, and many other body functions upon which we do not have direct control.

5. Practicing Yoga Improves Personal and Professional Relationships

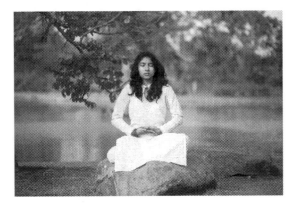

When your love, friendship, and other relationships are doing good, it's wonderful, but when they're bad, it's disastrous. Trouble in relationships may be caused by unhappiness, depression, low-self-esteem or sometimes, we also overburden the relationship with our wounds and pain we carry from our past.

The practise of yoga is a reliable resource for creating sustainable relationships. Practise of yoga empowers you to be your own healer. Through yoga we come to know and love ourselves, we find self-acceptance, and become self-aware, self-responsible, and self-loving. It makes you realise if we love ourselves, only then will we be in position to offer it to others. As you and your self-care, self-love grows, you will see that there will be an incredible change in your relationships. Often, the feelings of anger and hurt sit in our physical body, holding us back. Yoga helps us to find forgiveness and release them. When our inner world changes, we tend to see the reflection in the external world. Yoga practise seeds up the wish to make a purposeful difference on the planet.

To enter into personal transformation in a yogic way, the first two limbs of the eight-limbed path of yoga, the *Yamas* and *Niyamas*, are utmost beneficial.

The *Yamas* follow the five personal disciplines as *ahimsa* or non-violence, *satya* or truthfulness, *asteya* or non-stealing, *brahmacharya* or moderation, and *aparigraha* or non-grasping. Practising *ahimsa* will reflect the way you treat others and like to be treated.

The *Niyamas* are five personal disciplines more focused on how you treat yourself: *saucha* or cleanliness, *santosha* or contentment, *tapas* or discipline, *svadhyaya* or self-study, and *isvarapranidhana* or connection to the divine. Cultivating *Niyamas* in you will affect those around you in the sense how you behave around them and how they perceive you.

So don't delay. Roll your mat today, breathe deeply, strike a yoga pose, and watch your relationships bloom!

6. Yoga Benefits People Living with Depression

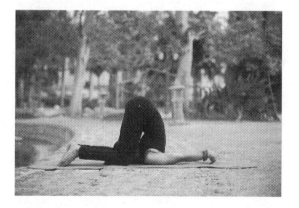

Depression is the price our generation pays in an age of constant digital bombardment. Anyone reading this will not agree if I say depression has become biggest killer after HIV! And only 14 per cent of people suffering from depression can be revived by medical treatment.

Studies and gurus are logical when they say that about 65 per cent of depression cases can be cured by yogic techniques. Yoga doesn't cure as a drug, but it transforms lives naturally. Here, it is where physical treatments end and psychological practises begin.

Yoga practise can vary from gentle to strenuous and challenging. The choice of style tends to be based on physical ability and personal preference, or the condition one wants to treat.

Mental and physical health are not just closely bonded, but also give almost zero results if attempted to address alone. The deep physiological state of rest induced by the three yogic elements of *yogasanas*, guided meditation, and controlled breathing for forty-five minutes six times in a week involving several types of cyclical patterns, ranging from slow and calming to rapid and stimulating, not only treats depression by 67 per cent but also the preliminary stage of any kind of an addiction.

Deep breathing and meditation does wonders for your mood by triggering the production of serotonin—the feeling of elation that comes from releasing built-up stress and emotion in your body. While performing *asanas*, there may be times when you feel uncomfortable, angry, or agitated, and you want to come out of a pose, but yoga teaches you to notice how you feel and to use your breath to accept your current discomfort and adjust. You'll learn that as quickly as sadness arises, it also fades away. Developing the ability to stay with pain will eventually subside it.

If your mind and energy are out of control, you're feeling agitated, anxious, and fearful; you might assume that it's depression.

Best *yogasana* practises for a depressed person would be:

1. Sun salutations (*surya namaskar*)
2. *Adho Mukha Svanasana* (downward-facing dog pose)
3. *Virbhadrasana* (warrior pose)
4. Paschimottanasana (seated forward bend)
5. *Balasana* (child's pose)
6. *Sarvangasana* (shoulder stand)
7. *Halasana* (plow pose)
8. *Chakrasana* (wheel pose)

Lastly, end on a positive note by lying in *Savasana* (corpse pose) for ten minutes.

7. Yoga Reduces the Risk of Heart Diseases

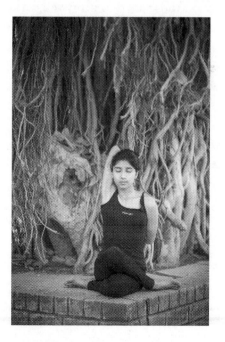

Yoga has a beneficial impact on heart's health just as exercises like jogging, brisk walking, or cycling have at relatively low cost. The biggest benefit of yoga is that it's easy to practise at home, doesn't require much space, is not weather dependent, and it can be practised by people who are physically inactive or those who are old and week.

People struggling with stressful or even physically inactive lifestyle and poor diet may have a higher risk for heart diseases, as it causes their heart to beat faster and their blood pressure also increases. This long-term high blood pressure can weaken their heart and damage blood vessels and narrow arteries. This is a leading cause of heart attack. So the cycle starts with stress, and yoga has ability to decrease the body's response to stress. Though yoga may not fully prevent or reverse a damaged system, but it will surely change it. And more the energy you put into it, more results you get.

What you need to do is look for a yoga class that includes the *Asanas*, breathing, meditation, and a trained instructor who can modify poses to meet your abilities and requirements. Practising various yoga as a therapy session for twelve weeks can lower blood pressure and cholesterol levels, improve heart rate and respiratory system, and also exercise and tone up the muscles. Anything that works your muscles is good for your blood vessels.

Most Effective Yoga Poses For Heart are:

Anuloma Vilomna Pranayama (alternate nostrils Breathing)

It fills your lungs with fresh oxygen, and is immensely powerful in relieving stress, which is one of the major causes of heart problems. Perform this *pranayama* by sitting cross-legged. Inhale deeply and gradually through your right nostril, while keeping your left nostril shut with the middle finger of your right hand. Exhale through your left nostril, while keeping your right nostril shut with your thumb. Keep repeating the cycle with alternate nostrils for fifteen to twenty times.

Brahmari Pranyama (humming the bee sound)

It relieves anger and anxiety, thus, relieving mental stress. Perform this *pranayama* by sitting cross-legged on the floor and closing your eardrums with your index fingers. Now, chant 'om' with your mouth, and let the internal sound vibrate your brain, buzzing of a bee.

Asanas for healthy heart:

1. *Pawanmuktasana* with right leg
2. *Goumukh asana*
3. *Setuband asana*
4. *Naukasana* (on back)
5. *Trikonasana*
6. *Virbhadrasana*
7. *Chakrasana*
8. *Uddiyan bandh*
9. *Tadasana*
10. *Vrikshasana*
11. *Ardhmatsyendra asana*
12. *Manjari asana*

Lastly, end on a positive note; lie in *Savasana* for ten minutes.

8. Eight Weeks of Regular Yoga Improves your Sleep
    Quality.

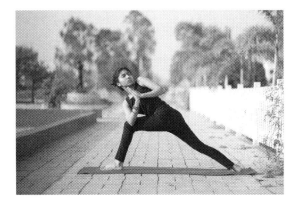

The only treasure that money can't buy is sleep. Factors causing lack of sleep may vary from change in one's sleeping environment, change of work shift, pain due to disease or illness, but major factors remain anxiety and depression. When your mind keeps wandering through thoughts or a long to-do list, it becomes hard to fall asleep. Older people are at higher risk for insomnia. Lack of good sleep results in mood swings, fatigue, low energy levels, frustration, lack of concentration, and lack of motivation. Lack of sleep in long term may result in obesity (weight gain), high blood pressure, and other cardiovascular problems.

Insomnia may be common, but if left untreated, its health consequences can cause disaster. Any treatment is best to begin with. Basic lifestyle changes and yoga and mindfulness meditation can be effective treatments for insomnia and other sleep disorders. It works by improving your sleeping patterns through exercise, and is especially effective for those who lead a relatively sedentary lifestyle.

Certain poses nourish tissues and nervous system and balance the hormones in your brain, thus, relaxing the whole system. An evening yoga practise can further add significantly to sleep efficiency.

Mindfulness Meditation

Practising mindfulness meditation for twenty minutes every day involves concentrating on your breathing, and then bringing your mind's attention to the present without racing into concerns about the past or future. If you cannot concentrate on your breath, choose a sound, preferably 'om' and keep chanting inside as you inhale and exhale. If at all your thoughts wander in between, don't worry, and start again with a deep breath return your focus returns to chanting.

Effective *asanas* to help you sleep:

1. *Utkatasana*
2. *Dhanur asana*
3. *Matsyasana*
4. *Ardhchandrasana*
5. *Tadasana*
6. *Kapotasana*
7. *Parivrtta Trikonasana*
8. *Vrkshasana*
9. *Manjari asana*
10. *Halasana*
11. *Parvatasana*

Lastly, end on a positive note; lie in *Savasana* for ten minutes.

9. meditation boosts memory

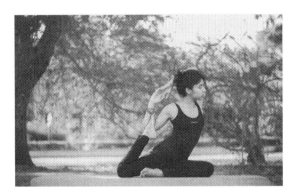

How easy it is to be glued to our favourite TV show or our favourite book without any effort but Imagine on a afternoon your teacher gruelling with a lesson of a subject you are not too fond of. You are sitting on a bench with the textbook open on the desk, but you are feeling lethargic, your mind is off on a trip. Poor concentration and forgetfulness is a common problem amongst we students, and it is worst when we need it most.

The pressure and stress of performance, peer conflicts and gadget challenges take a toll on the brain. This should be actual reason to inculcate 'Yoga' in our curriculum as proposed by our Yog enthusiast prime minister, because yog with its unique combination of postures, meditation and relaxation breathing, can be a great antidote to an epidemic of memory loss, stimulating the generation of new brain cells, which can then migrate from one area of the brain to another, and train the brain to work better. Yoga also keeps those new brain cells alive and active.

Meditation is all about increased and sustained concentration, 'making wandering mind wondering minds'.

It surely will help children to reduce thoughts in the mind, improves focus and performance. Excessive thinking consumes mental energy. For instance when you are feeling too anxious before an exam, a few minutes of meditating will help you collect your thoughts better and retain all that you have learnt, and would help you write your exam with a clearer calmer mind

Vrikshasana focuses mind so that you are not susceptible to the distractions and balances the emotions.

Also Postures like pashimottasana, Sarvangasana, Halasana, Matsyendrasana and Sun salutation help increase blood circulation and oxygen flow to the brain thus boosting memory and retention power and in other ways will give you deep physical and mental rest, which means a good goodnight sleep which will avoid you from feeling lethargic during lessons. Plan your time better and finish your studies in lesser time than you usually spent.

So basically, put down that gadget and pick up your mat!

10. Yoga to cure asthama

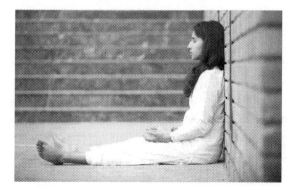

I belong to a family of marathoners, and my mother always wanted my Aunt to take part in marathons, but due to the fear of asthama attack she always denied!! There are many people who restrict themselves from even the slightest of exertion due to the fear of asthama. Yog is an effective solution for them. Specially breathing techniques can be the foundation for a asthama treatment.

Asthama is a very common respiratory complaint, which causes difficulty in breathing, specifically when breathing out. Because of the poor lung functioning, one cannot eliminate the entire carbon dioxide from the body during normal breathing.

Asthmatics should avoid:

1. Breathing exercises which call for rapid breathing like kapalbhati and bhastrika
2. Retention of the inhalation like antara kumbhaka
3. Tightening of the throat like ujjayi pranayama
4. Sun- Salutation as it takes a lot of strength and stamina to perform.

Keep sipping water to help keep your airways moist and breathe through your nose during all the exercises, as asthmatics are often mouth breathers.

Start with deep relaxation breathing

Remember to shorten inhalation to half of the exhalation. Inhale deeply and as you inhale make sure that your abdomen rises up and not your chest. And When you exhale feel your abdomen going down. Repeat 10 - 15 time followed by Nadi Shodhan pranayama (Alternate nostril breathing)

Then Practice postures that involve in expanding of chest, to increase breathing capacity of lungs like:

1. tadasana
2. Ustrasana
3. Ardha Matsyendrasana
4. Pavanamuktasana
5. Setu Bandh Asana
6. matsyasana
7. Adho Mukha Svanasana
8. uthitpadasana
9. Bhujangasana
10. shavasana

11. Hasyayoga proves, 'Laughter is the best medicine'

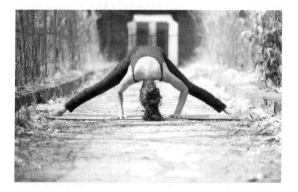

Laughter yoga (Hasyayoga) is a practice involving forced Laughter. This great discovery in Yog was done by an Indian, Dr. Madan Kataria. It is based on the belief that forced laughter incorporated with yogic breathing provides the same benefits as real laughter and brings more oxygen to the body and brain thus benefitting to cardiovascular health. Laughter indisputably breaks the cycle of psychological negative thinking, helping in releasing blocked emotions, depression or anger and boosts up the Mood and affects productivity. It also breaks down the inhibitions between people and enhances social bonding. Some studies also suggest that pain threshold becomes remarkably higher after laughter. In some prisons and jails, it's given as a rehabilitation therapy. World Laughter Day is now celebrated worldwide on the first Sunday of May of every year.

Laughter yoga is done in groups where participants do not need to have a good sense of humor, know jokes, or even be funny or happy. The idea is to "laugh for no reason"; one person laughing is enough to get the whole group to laugh and turn into real laughter. 'Laughter is contagious.'

Start the session with gentle warm-up activities like clapping upside down and chanting "ho ho, ha-ha-ha", moving in a circle facing each other and making a eye contact to break the ice and encourage childlike playfulness between participants. Include roaring like a lion with tongue fully out, mouth open, and hands stretched out like the paws.

Then few Breathing exercises should be done to prepare the lungs for laughter. This is extremely important because when you deepen your breath, you calm your body and when you calm your body, you calm your mind and start living in the present moment where you can experience happiness.

Now start laughter exercises to encourage laughter and joy like electric shock treatment, mad dancing, and pretending to do certain other activities. Chant "Very good, very good and "Yay" after every exercise swinging your arms upward and downward as you chant. The laughter should be loud and deep with arms stretched out towards the sky, head tilted back and chin raised up.

"We don't laugh because we are happy. We are happy because we laugh."

Reach out for a laughter session near you

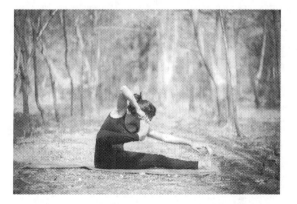

12. Shut migraine out of your life in 12 weeks

Whenever we asked my Mama(uncle) to accompany us to a hil station for holidays, his feets became cold in the fear of migraine, I have grown up realising his migraine was triggered with bright light, noise, sun glare, strong smell, stress, constipation, acidity,hunger or even chocolates!!! he has-been suffering from this neurological condition for years now.Migraine causes him unbearable pain Usually in one side of head. I really wanted to cure him before he reached the point where medicine was necessary.

there a natural way 'Yog' to make your resistance against migraine better by lessening the impact of a migraine attack. For migraine sufferers yoga promisingly improves blood circulation, calms down the nervous system,relaxes mind, reduces pain and anxiety, relieves stress and headache and gives you a good goodnight sleep.pranayama and meditation reduce the activities in the brain that lead to stress

Yoga is not that 'one size fits all'. In some cases of migraine sufferers find the situation worse in forward bending yoga postures!! Whereas in some cases the same postures miraculously treat the twenty year old migraine pain at once!! For some just pressing on top of ring finger,thumb and centre of palm of both hands worked wonderfully

In any yoga posture to cure migraine the head should not be lower than heart.

The regular practice of these Aasana for 12 weeks can help incredibly

1. Padmasana
2. Paschimottanasana
3. Adho Mukha Svanasana
4. Marjariasana
5. setubandhasana
6. Bhujang asana
7. kapaal bhati
8. Bhastrika
9. yoga nidra gives the best result. (YogaNidra is a state of conscious Deep Sleep. YogaNidra brings an incredible calmness and quietness)

Write to me at palak@palakgarg.in or gargpalak101199@gmail.com

Visit me on my website www.palakgarg.in
Check out my blog at www.palakgarg.in/blog
Follow me on Twitter www.twitter.com/@palakgarg99
Watch me performing at my YouTube channel
    -www.youtube.com/palakgarg
Find me on Facebook at www.facebook.com/palakgarg.in
Connect with me on Google+ at gargpalak99@gmail.com